JANUA LINGUARUM

STUDIA MEMORIAE
NICOLAI VAN WIJK DEDICATA

edenda curat

C. H. VAN SCHOONEVELD

Indiana University

Series Minor, 153

A PHONOLOGICAL INVESTIGATION OF APHASIC SPEECH

by

SHEILA E. BLUMSTEIN

Brown University
and
Aphasia Research Center, Boston

1973

MOUTON

THE HAGUE · PARIS

LIBRARY OF CONGRESS CATALOG CARD NUMBER: 72-94448

Printed in The Netherlands

ACKNOWLEDGEMENTS

This monograph is a revision of my doctoral dissertation in linguistics, Harvard University, 1970. Many people have been instrumental in bringing this study from its inception to completion as dissertation and finally in this revised and edited form. Special thanks to Eugene Green and D. Frank Benson of the Aphasia Research Unit, Veterans Administration Hospital, Boston; Frank Spellacy, University of Victoria; Susumu Kuno, Harvard University; and Hope Fisher, Brown University. My deepest gratitude goes to Roman Jakobson and Harold Goodglass both of whom demonstrated a profound interest in this research investigation in every stage of its development. Their invaluable criticism, assistance and advice helped clarify many of the problems encountered in this study. It is to them that this monograph is dedicated.

This work was supported in part by pre-doctoral NIH Fellowship 2 FO1 MH 40094-02 MTLH and USPHS Grants NS 07615 to Clark University and NS 06209 to Boston University.

PREFACE

Aphasia is a disorder of language produced by injury to the brain structures most essential for language functioning. Thus, by definition, it would seem to be an area in which linguistic analysis of the defects should make a contribution, at least at a descriptive level. However, as one surveys the varied but recurring patterns of language disturbance and their relationship to the specific site of brain injury, the relevance of linguistic techniques of study becomes even more compelling. One discovers that, depending on the structures damaged, there may be conspicuous symptoms at the level of phonology, in the area of lexicon, or in the area of syntax. These linguistic levels are not of course the final explanation of the underlying defect. One task of the psycholinguistic researcher is to explicate the psychological processes which are manifested in, for example, a selective loss of concept naming by a patient whose articulation and grammar are intact. Turning to the structures whose injury produces this defect, and utilizing both neuroanatomical and behavioral evidence as to the role their structures play in the brain, one may begin to infer the mechanisms of the psychological processes which produce a selective disorder. Linguistic analysis provides potentially fruitful means of examining the dimensions of the disorder.

Just as the linguist may help detect those features of aphasic disorder which are a critical clue to understanding brain function, so may the phenomena of aphasia provide tests of the validity of certain aspects of linguistic theory. This is most obvious with respect to those theories which predict the order of complexity or degrees of relationship among performances in the same general sphere. For example, if an aphasic patient is most disturbed in syntax, do the observed order of difficulty of syntactic structures, and the observed clustering of types of errors conform to syntactic theory? If not, perhaps they suggest alternative explanations which may be relevant to normal language.

Dr. Blumstein has approached the problem of phonology from both of the points of view outlined here: (1) to see how the linguistic analysis of the phonologic defects improves the clinical description of the patient's disorder, and consequently reflects on the function of the affected brain structures; (2) to see whether theoretical linguistic predictions as to the order of difficulty and the order of relatedness of phonological performance is supported by the natural phenomenon of aphasia.

As a psychologist and clinician, rather than a linguist, I will address myself principally to the importance of the first of these goals. It is generally agreed among aphasiologists that injuries to the anterior portion of the left hemisphere speech area are most commonly associated with disorders of articulation – e.g., with inability to direct the speech apparatus in the correct formation or ordering of English sounds. In some instances, speech movements are so laborious and awkward that, at best, the sounds uttered are clumsy approximations of the intended phonemes. In other cases, individual phonemes are easily and correctly produced but their choice and sequential ordering is affected. The contemporary French aphasiologists refer to these two types as disorders at the 'phonetic' vs. the 'phonemic' level. In still another group of patients the disordered selection and sequencing of sounds and syllables appears to be part of a broader disorder in which the inner acoustic image of the word is weakened along with precision in selection of intended words. In the latter group of patients (Wernicke aphasics) familiar motor speech sequences seem to run uncontrolled, with neologisms, word substitutions, and contaminations from one word to another. Thus, phoneme substitutions occurring in this context might well be presumed to follow different rules from those which seem to be the product of poor motor control.

Still another possible mechanism which might be thought to influence phonological output in a particular way is the impaired execution of any purposeful movements (i.e., apraxia) of the articulatory apparatus – even for such non-speech actions as licking lips, blowing, or coughing. While some investigators believe that articulatory difficulties are the RESULT of the underlying apraxia, there is evidence, too, that these are parallel, but not causally related phenomena.

It is obvious, then, that a comparison is needed of the various groups of speech disordered patients, from the point of view of the phonological rules which predict their errors. The demonstration that phonological rules of different sorts characterized their errors would give us a foothold in differentiating between the clinical types. On the other hand, uniformity in the operation of the rules might indicate that there are common principles determining articulatory errors which are unaffected by the clinical differences which have been described.

Dr. Blumstein has carried out a complex task with great objectivity. Her approach brings to bear on the problem the best that is currently known about clinical diagnosis in aphasia, sophisticated application of linguistic theory, and the appropriate use of statistical techniques. The result is a significant contribution both to aphasiology and to linguistic theory of phonology.

HAROLD GOODGLASS, PH. D.
Professor of Neuropsychology
Director, Boston University
Aphasia Research Center

TABLE OF CONTENTS

PART II

IMPLICATIONS FOR PHONOLOGICAL THEORY

LIST OF FIGURES

LIST OF TABLES

LIST OF SYMBOLS

Consonants

Standard IPA: *p*, *t*, *k*, *b*, *d*, *g*, *f*, *s*, *v*, *z*, *m*, *n*, *r*, *l*, *w*, *y*, *h*

θ as in *th*ink
ð as in *th*e
š as in *sh*eep
ž as in bei*g*e
č as in *ch*air
ǰ as in *j*ug
ŋ as in si*ng*
ʔ as in moun*t*ain
ɾ as in Be*tt*y
ṛ as in b*ir*d
ṇ as in butt*on*
ḷ as in midd*le*

Vowels

Standard IPA: *i*, *e*, *a*, *o*, *u*

I as in b*i*t
E as in b*e*t
æ as in b*a*t
ɔ as in b*ough*t
ə as in b*u*t
U as in b*oo*k

INTRODUCTION

The following study is an experimental investigation of the phonological patterns of aphasic speech. It is the object of this study to characterize the patterns of phonological dissolution and to consider the implications of the results obtained for aphasiology, on the one hand, and linguistic theory, on the other.

As an interdisciplinary investigation, some issues will be discussed which are completely new to either the aphasiologist or the linguist. Others will be of only secondary interest to either one of the disciplines. Consequently, this monograph is divided into two parts.

The first part deals with the experimental aspects of the study with emphasis on methodology, preliminary bases, and statistical analyses. The results are discussed in relation to the field of aphasia. Specifically, we hope to compare the speech patterns of different clinical types of aphasia and discuss the similarities and differences of the patterns underlying each clinical syndrome.

In the second part, we are concerned with the theoretical linguistic issues raised by an analysis of the aphasic data. We hope to examine the validity of the phonological framework on the basis of empirical evidence, discuss the theoretical problems encountered in the analysis, and suggest possible alternative solutions.

The first chapter of the monograph is essential to members of both disciplines. It places the investigation in its historical perspective, introduces the reader to the theoretical linguistic framework as well as the clinical types of aphasia, and attempts to integrate all of these aspects in the presentation of the study's objectives.

PART I

PHONOLOGICAL ANALYSIS OF APHASIC SPEECH

1

THEORETICAL AND HISTORICAL PERSPECTIVES

One of the primary goals of linguistic research is to develop a theory of language which will specify the theoretical constructs underlying linguistic systems and characterize their inter-relationships. Empirical verification of linguistic theories is of obvious necessity. In the pathology of language, aphasia, many aspects of the linguistic code break down along specifiable parameters. For this reason, the study of aphasia may give insights into the structure of these parameters and their subsequent organization into the unity-language.

It has been commonly observed in clinical testing that the speech pattern of aphasics contains many types of phonological errors. Paul Broca's first description of aphasia in 1863 focused on the loss of articulatory capacity due to impairment of "la mémoire des moyens de co-ordination que l'on emploie pour articuler les mots".[1] In the ensuing sixty years, aphasiologists such as Hughlings Jackson, E. Fröschels, H. Head, and K. Goldstein frequently cited instances of phonemic errors in the speech output of certain types of aphasic patients.[2] These observations, however, were made in the context of diagnostic descriptions of aphasic syndromes. There was no concept of the phonological system as a linguistic organization, and thus, no systematic study of phonological errors.

[1] P. Broca, *Extraits des Bulletins de la Société Anatomique*, 1863, quoted in *Selected Writings of John Hughlings Jackson*, II, ed. J. Taylor (New York, 1958).

[2] c.f. J. H. Jackson, *Selected Writings*, II (New York, 1958); E. Fröschels, "Zur behandlung des motorischen aphasie", *Archives Psychiatrist*, 56, 1–19 (1915); H. Head, *Aphasia and Kindred Disorders of Speech*, I-II (New York, 1926); and K. Goldstein, *Language and Language Disturbances* (New York, 1948).

After 1925 several systematic studies were conducted expressly to ascertain the nature of these phonological errors.[3] Although using different methodologies including repetition and reading of nonsense and/or real words, full sentences and paragraphs, the investigators made very similar observations. Firstly, similar types of phonological errors seemed to be made by the aphasic patients. These errors included – the substitution of one phoneme for another, addition and loss of phonemes, and improper sequencing of phonemes. Moreover, all noted that phoneme substitution errors seemed to occur among 'similar' phonemes, i.e. voiced and voiceless consonants were substituted for each other, nasals and their homorganic stops were confused, spirants and stops were varied.[4]
Some examples of these types of errors are:

/dei/'day' → /tei/ $C_{voiced} \rightarrow C_{voiceless}$

/sop/'soap' → /top/ $C_{spirant} \rightarrow C_{stop}$

[3] c.f. I. Bouman and A. Grünbaum, "Experimentell-psychologische untersuchungen zur aphasie und paraphasie", *Zeitschrift für die gesamte Neurologie und Psychiatrie*, 96, 481–538 (1925); A. Ombredane, "Sur le mécanisme de l'anarthrie", *Journal de Psychologie Normale et Pathologique*, 61, 940–955 (1926); T. Alajouanine, A. Ombredane and M. Durand, *Le Syndrome de la Désintégration Phonétique dans l'Aphasie* (Paris, 1939); D. B. Fry, "Phonemic substitutions in an aphasic patient", *Language and Speech*, 2, 52–56 (1959); D. Cohen, J. Dubois, M. Gauthier, H. Hécaen and R. Angelergues, "Aspects du fonctionnement du code linguistique chez les aphasiques moteurs", *Neuropsychologia*, 1, 165–177 (1963); D. Shankweiler and K. Harris, "An experimental approach to the problem of articulation in aphasia", *Cortex*, 2, 277–292 (1966).

[4] To be sure not all investigators have accepted the conclusion that the phonological disintegration of aphasic speech is systematic or predictable (c.f. M. Critchley, "Articulatory defects in aphasia", *Journal of Laryngology and Otology*, 66, 1–17 (1952) 11ff.; Shankweiler and Harris, "Articulation in aphasia", 289ff.; R. Tikofsky, *Phonetic Characteristics of Dysarthria*, (Ann Arbor, 1965) 44, 65. Several have emphasized the variability of patient performance from day to day as well as the impossibility of predicting specific phonological errors. Variability in performance is not directly at issue in considering the phonological patterns underlying aphasic performance; i.e. although the quantity of errors may in fact vary from day to day, the direction and types of errors should remain qualitatively similar. Moreover, phonological theory in no way attempts to predict the specific occurrence of an error at any one time. Rather, it specifies the theoretical directions any error may take based on phonological principles underlying the language system.

/kiŋ/'king' → /tiŋ/ $C_{back} \rightarrow C_{front}$

The results of these studies suggested to us that there was an underlying uniformity in the phonological patterns of these patients and that this uniformity could be characterized simply and insightfully by the distinctive feature framework discussed by Jakobson, Halle, and Fant.[5] Briefly, this theory states that every phoneme can be described in terms of a bundle of binary acoustic-articulatory features. Every phoneme is characterized by the minimum number of features needed to differentiate it from all the phonemes within a given system; for example, the only feature needed to distinguish /d/ from /n/ is nasal; /d/ is [− nasal] and /n/ is [+ nasal]. Implicit in this theory is the notion that phonemes differentiated by a single feature are more closely aligned structurally, motorically and acoustically, as well as psychologically than phonemes separated by several features. For example, the relationship between d-n, distinguished by the feature [nasal], is closer than d-m, distinguished by the features $\begin{bmatrix}\text{nasal}\\\text{place}\end{bmatrix}$. Consequently, it would be expected that in the phonological dissolution of aphasic speech, the number of substitution errors would decrease as the phonological distance between phonemes increased. Thus, more substitution errors should occur between those phonemes separated by one distinctive feature, and fewer errors should occur between those phonemes separated by two distinctive features.

According to phonological theory, these distinctive features used to define phonemic relationships do not have equal value within the system. Rather, they are hierarchically organized. This notion was first introduced by Jakobson in his comparative analysis of the acquisition and dissolution of language in relation to phonological linguistic theory.[6] Implicit in his discussion of a phonological hierarchy were two important concepts – (1) the principle of maximal contrast which stated that the hierarchical relationships between sounds progressed from simple and undifferentiated to

[5] *Preliminaries to speech analysis* (Cambridge, 1962).

[6] *Child Language, Aphasia and Phonological Universals* (The Hague, 1968) 46 ff., 68 ff.

stratified and differentiated; (2) the law of implication which stated that the acquisition (and dissolution) of one phoneme implied the earlier command (loss) of a different phoneme. For example, the acquisition of affricates implied the previous acquisition of stops and fricatives; inversely, the loss of fricatives in aphasia implied the loss of affricates. The consonantal hierarchy postulated by Jakobson is stated informally below:

labial-dental stops
front-back stops
fricatives
affricates
laterals-resonants

Several studies on the phonology of aphasic speech have proposed a hierarchy of features based on the number and types of substitution errors made by aphasic patients.[7] A comparison of these hierarchies reveals a few discrepancies. Compare:

manner	place
place	manner
voice	voice
nasality	nasality

Because each investigation was based on a different feature framework and because not all of the tests devised included all possible consonants and their environmental positions, it is impossible to freely compare the hierarchies established. Nevertheless the similarities between the hierarchies proposed suggest that the features characterizing the phonological system are differentially but systematically affected. Consequently, it was felt that a systematic analysis of one distinctive feature substitution errors may give further insights into the underlying organization of the distinctive feature system.

Phonological theory is not only concerned with the notion distinc-

[7] Fry, "Phonemic substitutions", 57; S. Blumstein, "Phonological aspects of aphasic speech", in *Studies Presented to Professor R. Jakobson by his Students*, ed. C. Gribble (Cambridge, 1968) 41.

tive feature, but it is also concerned with the notion markedness, and ultimately the nature of the relationship between these two concepts. Before considering markedness in relation to the phonology of aphasic speech, the general theoretical basis of this notion will be briefly reviewed. Since its inception in the 1930's, markedness has become of increasing importance in linguistic theory and analysis, and in particular in phonology. Markedness was first defined by Trubetzkoy in *Gründzuge der Phonologie* to characterize the relationship between the values of one type of phonological opposition – the privative opposition. "Privative Oppositionen sind solche, bei denen das eine Oppositionsglied durch das Vorhandensein, das andere durch das Nichtvorhandensein eines Merkmales gekennzeichnet sind, z.B. 'stimmhalf'-'stimmlos', 'nasaliert'-'unnasaliert', ... Das Oppositionsglied, das durch das Vorhandsein des Merkmals gekennzeichnet ist, heisst 'merkmaltragend', das durch das Fehlen des Merkmals gekennzeichnete Oppositionsglied 'merkmallos' ...".[8]

Rather than restricting binary distinctions to a small class of phonemes, Jakobson extended binary oppositions to all phonological distinctions in the system.[9] In this way, the notion markedness could be considered in relation to the entire phonological system. It is based on Jakobson's re-evalution of the phonological system that the notion of markedness has been developed in current phonological theory.

Essentially, markedness does more than define the presence or absence of a given feature in a phonemic opposition. It characterizes the hierarchical relationship between the phonemes based on the $\{\pm\}$ values of the features used to describe them. Thus, the unmarked member of a phonological opposition represents the more basic or 'natural' value while the addition of a marked value adds a new specification or complexity to the system. For example, the relationship between /d/ and /n/ is characterized by the absence of

[8] N. S. Trubetzkoy, *Grundzüge der Phonologie* (Gottingen, 1958), 67.
[9] c.f. "Observations sur le classement phonologiques des consonnes", in *Selected Writings*, I. (The Hague, 1962), 273 and R. Jakobson and M. Halle, *Fundamentals of Language* (The Hague, 1956), 44 ff.

nasality in the former ([– nasal]), and the presence of nasality ([+nasal]) in the latter. The addition of nasality complicates the articulatory mechanism in speech production such that a double resonator, the oral and nasal cavity, is needed in the production of a nasal consonant. In the production of an oral stop, on the other hand, only a single resonator, the oral cavity, is needed.

The criteria used to determine the marked and unmarked values for phonemes and the features comprising them include[10]: (1) internal evidence within the phonological system of the language based on examples of neutralization – in the position of neutralization, the unmarked variant occurs more frequently than the marked variant; (2) evidence from historical linguistics – the loss of markedness values in historical phonology is more typical of marked variants than unmarked variants; (3) physiological and perceptual investigations – marked values present added complexities to production or perception; (4) evidence from acquisition of language – the more basic phonological distinctions are learned first by the child, while the more marked values are learned later; (5) evidence based on frequency factors within the language system – there are never more marked contrasts than unmarked contrasts within any given system. In addition, unmarked phonemes tend to have a greater frequency of occurrence than marked phonemes; (6) evidence from linguistic universals – in universal implicational statements of phonology, the unmarked feature is always implied. Moreover, the features common to most languages are the unmarked values; and finally, (7) evidence based on pathological language disturbance – the phonological dissolution of aphasic speech should be characterized by a tendency for the marked structures to be impaired in relation to the relative preservation of the unmarked structures.[11]

[10] For a detailed discussion of these criteria see J. Greenberg, "Language universals", in *Current Trends in Linguistics*, III, ed. T. Sebeok (The Hague, 1966) 62 ff.; R. Jakobson, "Implications of language universals for linguistics", in *Universals of Language*, ed. J. Greenberg (Cambridge, 1963) 265; P. Postal, *Aspects of Phonological Theory* (New York, 1968) 168 ff.

[11] R. Jakobson, "Linguistic types of aphasia", in *Brain Function*, III, ed. E. Carterette (California, 1963) 71 ff.; Blumstein, "Phonological aspects", 41.

The positing of phonological structures bound by relations intrinsic to the language system in particular and language structure in general has important theoretical consequences with regard to aphasia proper. For it implies, that regardless of the different clinical types of aphasia and their different underlying pathologies, that the phonological dissolution of speech will be directed by the same linguistic principles – namely, errors between phonemes related by one distinctive feature should occur more frequently than phonemes related by more than one distinctive feature; the feature hierarchy should be similarly affected; and marked structures should be more impaired than unmarked structures.

All the studies discussed thus far have been limited to patients with anterior or subcortical lesions. Luria noted that among the various linguistic difficulties noted in the so-called fluent aphasics, i.e. patients with posterior lesions, that phonemic substitutions or 'phonematic' disintegration was a common characteristic.[12] Systematic phonological studies of these types of aphasics have all noted features similar to those described by the investigations of patients with anterior lesions.[13] These features include phoneme substitution errors, errors of addition and simplification, and errors involving the proper sequencing of phonemes.

Although Blumstein compared the speech pattern of a fluent aphasic with the results described by Alajouanine et al.,[14] no systematic comparison of the phonological patterns of different clinical types of aphasics has been undertaken using the same methodology and theoretical premises. Consequently, three distinct aphasic groups will be considered in this study – Broca's, Conduction,

[12] "The pathology of directive function of speech", *Reports at the VIIth International Congress of Neurology* (Rome, 1961) 601 ff.

[13] c.f. V. W. Schenk, "Troubles des phonèmes en cas d'aphasie sensorielle", *Encéphale*, 42, 158–169 (1953); J. Dubois, H. Hécaen, R. Angelergues, M. Chatelier, P. Marcie, "Etudes neurolinguistiques de l'aphasie de conduction", *Neuropsychologia*, 2, 9–44 (1964); A. R. Lecours and F. Lhermitte, "Phonemic paraphasias: linguistic structures and tentative hypotheses", *Cortex*, 5, 193–228 (1969); E. Green, "Phonological and grammatical aspects of jargon in an aphasic patient: a case study", *Language and Speech*, 12, 103–118 (1969).

[14] c.f. Blumstein; Alajouanine et al.

and Wernicke's aphasics.[15] Each aphasic group can be distinguished by distinct clinical characteristics and accompanying pathology.

Broca's aphasia has been described as a contiguity disorder or expressive disorder of language.[16] Words which rely on surrounding context as articles, pronouns, and connectives are commonly omitted resulting in so-called 'telegraphic' speech. The speech production of these aphasics, often described as dysarthric, is characterized by slow, slurred production, frequent phonetic errors, distorted intonation patterns, and often difficulty in initiating speech. Comprehension and naming are usually intact or mildly impaired while errors in repetition are either less than or of approximately the same magnitude as spontaneous speech. The brain damage resulting in this syndrome is localized in the third frontal convolution (anterior section) of the speech area (see Figure 1).[17] Many researchers have emphasized the dysarthric quality of speech typical of these aphasics and described the phonology of these patients in terms of 'phonetic disintegration'.[18] Thus, although there is no damage to the articulatory apparatus itself, i.e. the tongue, lips, palate, vocal cords, etc., there is great difficulty in articulating speech sounds correctly .Three principles were postulated by Alajouanine et al. to account for this syndrome: (1) paralytic – articulatory weakness; (2) dystonic – articulatory movements excessive in force and duration; (3) apraxic – gross difficulty in forming articulatory movements to command and some difficulty upon imitation.[19] These observations were supported by further spectographic analyses of aphasic speech.[20]

Dysarthric speech can be characterized by two distinct types of

[15] The system of classification has been devised by the research team at the Aphasia Research Center, Veterans Administration Hospital, Boston.

[16] R. Jakobson, "Towards a linguistic typology of aphasic impairments", in *Disorders of Language*, ed. A.V. S. de Reuck (Boston, 1964), 25 ff.

[17] Aphasic disturbances are rarely limited to cortical lesions. The role and extent of subcortical brain damage to language pathology has not been clearly determined. Consequently, discussion will be limited to cortical lesions.

[18] c.f. Alajouanine et al., *Le Syndrome* (1939).

[19] *Le Syndrome*, 118 ff.

[20] c.f. Tikofsky, *Phonetic Characteristics* and I. Lehiste, *Some Acoustic Characteristics of Dysarthria* (Switzerland, 1968).

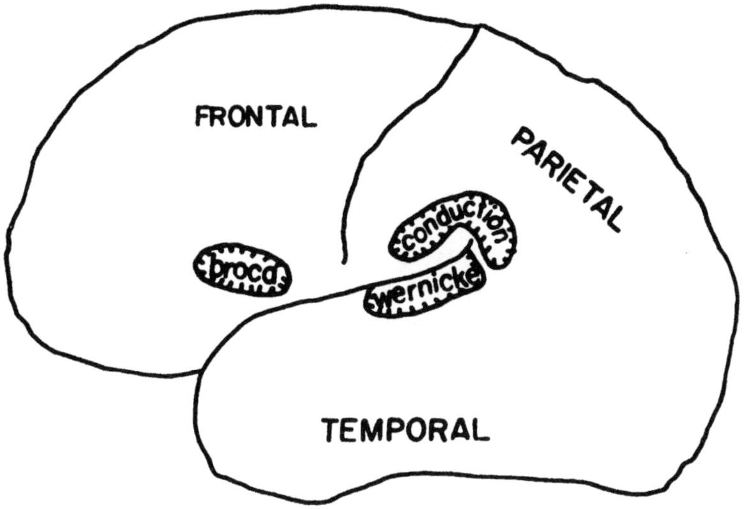

Fig. 1. Left cerebral cortex: Lesions producing aphasic syndromes

errors – (1) phonetic errors: those errors which either are so distorted phonetically that they are not definable as English phonemes or which modify only the articulatory production of a phoneme without affecting its phonemic value; (2) phonemic errors: those errors which clearly affect the distinctive values of the phonemes of the language. Because this study is limited only to the phonological patterns of aphasic speech, i.e. those patterns affecting the distinctive values of the system, only the latter type of error will be considered.

The dysarthric speech characteristic of Broca's aphasia is not found in Wernicke's or Conduction aphasia. These two syndromes are characterized by fluent speech with normal intonation and motor co-ordination.

Patients with Conduction aphasia commonly have good to excellent comprehension, poor repetition in relation to comprehension facility and fluent speech, and some naming difficulties. Spontaneous speech is interspersed with many examples of phonemic substitutions (literal paraphasias) and fewer instances of the substitution of one lexical item for another (verbal paraphasias).

The brain damage resulting in this syndrome is localized in the arcuate fasciculus.[21] This band of commissural fibers is considered to be the bridge between Wernicke's (posterior) and Broca's (anterior) area (see Figure 1).

Wernicke's aphasia, on the other hand, is characterized by impaired naming, repetition, and comprehension in the presence of fluent speech. Because selective operations as word finding are impaired, the spontaneous speech pattern of these patients is markedly circumlocutory and void of specific semantic content. Often patients produce a copious amount of verbal material and have marked difficulty in inhibiting this press for speech. Substitutions of one lexical item for another commonly occur. Some Wernicke's aphasics produce sequences of phonemes which can not be identified as English words. The amount of this neologistic jargon varies with each patient – some have neologisms interspersed in the prosodic sequence and others have complete phrases or sentences which can not be defined as meaningful English. The brain damage resulting in this syndrome is localized in the first temporal gyrus (see Figure 1). A review of the clinical features of these aphasic groups can be seen in Table 1.

TABLE 1

The Clinical Manifestations of Broca's, Conduction, and Wernicke's Aphasia

	Broca	Conduction	Wernicke
Spontaneous Sp. Fluent	−	+	+
Dysarthria	+	−	−
Comprehension	+	+	−
Naming	+	−	−
Repetition	±	−	−

As indicated earlier, phoneme substitution errors form only a small part of the total types of errors characteristic of the phonological patterns of aphasic patients. Thus, it is necessary to analyze these

[21] N. Geschwind, "Disconnexion syndromes in animals and man", II, *Brain*, 88, 585–644 (1965), 620.

other types of phonological errors and consider their relationship to the systematic disorganization of speech. If the organization of the phonemes of the language are hierarchically based, then it may indeed be the case that the types of errors made reflect a given order of difficulty. This notion and its implications for aphasia will be explored in depth.

In summary, there are three overall objectives in this investigation: (1) to determine the significant error categories comprising the phonological patterns of aphasic speech, and subsequently, to characterize them in some systematic way; (2) to explore the relationships, if any, between patterns of breakdown and different areas of brain pathology; and (3) to test theoretical linguistic assumptions on the basis of evidence from aphasia.

2

METHODOLOGY

2.1. SUBJECTS

The aphasia population represented in this study was drawn from three diagnostic groups – Broca, Conduction, and Wernicke aphasics. The classifications made were based on a composite aphasia examination including psychological, language, and neurological tests presented and discussed at the Aphasia Rounds of the Boston Veterans Administration Hospital Aphasia Research Unit. One patient's case was evaluated at the Boston University Medical School by the same diagnostic team.

There were no restrictions made in choice of patients based on etiology. Consequently, the sample consisted of subjects with brain damage resulting from trauma, vascular disease, or tumors.

In all, 17 subjects were included in this study – 6 Broca's, 5 Conduction, and 6 Wernicke's. There were 16 men and 1 woman ranging in age from 22 to 78 years, with a mean age of 53.2 years. No subject was examined until at least eight-weeks after onset of aphasia. The average number of years in school for this population was 12.5 with a range in education from eight grade through medical school. Occupations varied from housewife and itinerant worker to professional musician and practicing physician. Table 2 summarizes the significant features of each case.

TABLE 2

Patient Summary

Patient	Sex	Age	Education	Work	Etiology	Aphasia
J.D.	M	22	H.S.	none	trauma	Broca
A.S.	M	40	Master's Degree	H.S. math teacher	vascular	Broca
L.C.	M	49	9	prison guard	vascular	Broca
A.B.	M	50	9	shipper, chef	suspect vascular	Broca
P.B.	M	25	college	none	trauma	Broca
F.G.	M	71	Master's Degree	school teacher	vascular	Broca
W.B.	M	55	H.S.	machinist, metal worker	vascular	Conduction
A.K.	M	50	H.S.	career army, paratrooper	vascular	Conduction
E.S.	M	60	9	carpenter	suspect vascular	Conduction
M.J.	M	73	H.S.	V.A. job placement	vascular	Conduction
W.W.	M	50	H.S.	postal foreman	vascular	Conduction
F.C.	M	56	H.S.	unknown	vascular	Wernicke
A.G.	M	73	medical school	physician	vascular	Wernicke
L.K.	M	62	H.S., music school	entertainer, piano	tumor	Wernicke
T.C.	M	35	H.S.	stock boy	trauma	Wernicke
A.S.	M	78	8	fireman	vascular	Wernicke
E.K.	F	55	H.S.	housewife	vascular	Wernicke

2.2. TEST MATERIAL

The raw data for this study was obtained by conducting interviews with the aphasic patients. The test consisted of an open-ended conversation concerning the patients' illness, work, hobbies, view of politics, etc. Questions asked were used only as a means of eliciting as much speech as possible. Examples of questions used are found in Table 3.

Each sample consisted of a minimum of 2000 words. The size of each sample was determined by calculating the number of words said in four consecutive minutes and then estimating the necessary interview time necessary to reach the minimum word rate. Function words, connectives, and forms of the copula were not included in the word count. Clinical observations have shown that phonological errors in aphasic speech commonly occur on the content words and rarely on the function words. Moreover, because Broca's aphasics often eliminate these words, their sample consists predominantly of content words. Fluent aphasics, on the other hand, use these grammatical words in their speech. Consequently, a tabulation consisting of every word used by the patients would not give an equal chance of error for each aphasic group.

The object of this test was to obtain a corpus of material representative of the patient's speech output. This corpus, demonstrating the 'natural speech flow' of each patient, made possible the analysis of phonological errors in relation to the various phonological contexts in which they occurred. Moreover, the use of free speech interviews avoided many of the difficulties in interpretation presented by tasks 'forcing' a specific linguistic response. With these tests, it is impossible to determine whether the patient's performance is a direct result of the competence of his input mechanism (comprehension of the task or individual test item), his storage mechanism (retaining the item long enough to respond to it), his speech output mechanism, or an interaction of the three (contamination of the speech output with the input message). With the corpus limited to free speech utterances, it is possible to interpret a patient's errors as the result of the linguistic

TABLE 3

Examples of Interview Questions

(I) Hospital
- (a) how are you feeling?
- (b) what brought you into the hospital?
- (c) what is your main trouble?
- (d) what do you do in a day at the hospital?
- (e) how is the food? what did you have for breakfast? . . . etc.

(II) Family
- (a) are you married? for how long?
- (b) do you have any children?
  - (1) names, ages.
  - (2) what kinds of things do you do with them?

(III) Education (Depends on age of patient)
- (a) how far did you go in school?
- (b) what was your best subject? worst?

(IV) Employment
- (a) what kind of work did you do? describe it.
- (b) ask questions specifically on response, e.g. special training, etc.

(V) Hobbies
- (a) do you have any hobbies?
- (b) describe it (them).

(VI) Entertainment
- (a) do you like to read?
  - 1. books, magazines, newspapers?
  - 2. describe your favorite book, magazine, etc.
- (b) do you like T.V.?
  - 1. what shows do you watch?
  - 2. describe one of them.
- (c) do you like movies?
  - 1. what kinds do you like? describe one of them.
- (d) do you like sports? which ones?
  - 1. how do you play______?

(VII) Current Events

(VIII) Travel Experience
- (a) have you done any travelling?
- (b) where?

system and specifically the phonological system available to him for speech output.

2.3. EXPERIMENTAL PROCEDURE

Each patient was individually tested in a moderately quiet room. The entire session was recorded on a Uher 4000 Report L tape recorder. Spontaneous speech interviews lasted approximately 30-50 minutes. In the early sessions, the interviews were not held continuously but were interrupted with other activities for approximately 10-15 minutes duration. No testing session exceeded 50 minutes in length. Consequently, for all patients, several interview sessions were conducted, usually on successive days. If a patient indicated that he was tired, the session was terminated for the day. The number of test sessions varied from 2-9. This range can be accounted for by the nature of the clinical groups used in the study. The Broca's aphasics, who are characteristically non-fluent in verbal output, needed many more interviews to reach the minimum corpus size desired than the fluent (Conduction and Wernicke's) aphasics.

2.4. ANALYSIS OF DATA

The raw data used for this study was selected from the taped interviews. Each interview was listened to completely, and those phonological errors made by the patients were transcribed using the International Phonetic Alphabet. The attempted target word was also noted. Only those errors whose target words could clearly be determined by the surrounding context were used in the analysis. Those questionable items eliminated came from four sources: (1) where the surrounding context did not provide enough information to identify the target word. For example, in the sentence 'I saw a /læt/', it is impossible to determine if the patient wanted to say /kæt/ 'cat', /ræt/ 'rat', /næt/ 'gnat', and consequently, whether the phoneme substitution was $\left\{\begin{matrix}k\\r\\n\end{matrix}\right\} \rightarrow 1$; (2) where the item produced by the patient was so distorted phonetically that it bore no similarity to an English word. These examples are found predominantly in patients with dysarthric speech; (3) where the sequence produced by the patient bore no phonemic similarity to the target word which could ostensibly fit into the surrounding context, e.g. 'I went to a /tufbei/ party', target word is 'birthday'. This error is often called a neologism or jargon episode and is commonly found in the speech output of Wernicke's aphasics; (4) where the word produced by the patient was an obvious substitution of one word for another, e.g. /tiθ/ 'teeth' instead of /tið/ 'teethe'. This error type is commonly called a verbal paraphasia.

After all transcriptions were completed, the errors were classified into the following general categories:

Error type
(A) phoneme substitution
(B) simplification
(C) addition
(D) environment

The analysis first dealt with the various categories of error types:

(A) PHONEME SUBSTITUTION – These errors are characterized by the substitution of one phoneme for another, e.g. /timz/ 'teams' → /kimz/, /taim/ 'time' → /tain/.

(B) SIMPLIFICATION – These errors are characterized by the loss of a phoneme or syllable in a word. These two types of simplification were analyzed separately; e.g. phoneme simplification, /prIti/ 'pretty' → /pIti/, /frEnč/ 'French' → /fEnč/; syllable simplification, /EkspEnsIv/ 'expensive' → /pEnsIv/, /Emplɔiyə/ 'employer' → /plɔiyə/.

(C) ADDITION – As in (B), this category was divided into two subcategories – the addition of an extra phoneme or a syllable in a word, e.g. addition of a phoneme, /papa/ 'papa' → /papra/,

/əðəwaiz/ 'otherwise' → /əlðəwaiz/; addition of a syllable, e.g. /hElp/ 'help' → /hEləp/, /dIčt/ 'ditched' → /dəlIčt/.

(D) ENVIRONMENT – This classification included errors of phonemic substitutions which can be accounted for by the influence of surrounding phonemes. These errors are divided into 3 types:

(1) INTRA-MORPHEMIC BLENDS – a phonemic substitution triggered by a phoneme located in the same word. This assimilation may occur in anticipation of a given phoneme (regressive assimilation), e.g. /krit/ 'Crete' → /trit/, or by the contamination of an already occurring phoneme (progressive assimilation), e.g. /čæmpiənšIps/ 'championships' → /čæčInšIps/.

(2) INTER-MORPHEMIC BLENDS – errors triggered by phonemes or syllables located in neighboring words, e.g. /rost bif/ 'roast beef' → /rof bif/, /ai θiŋk so/ 'I think so' → /ai siŋk so/. These errors were also sub-categorized into errors of progressive and regressive assimilation.

(3) METATHESIS – errors characterized by the inversion of the order of phonemes in a given sequence, e.g. /dəgriz/ 'degrees' → /gədriz/, /ɔstrælia/ 'Australia' → /ɔtsrælia/.

In order to determine if specific phonological contexts triggered certain error types, the contexts in which each type of error occurred were analyzed. The contextual categories included all contexts in which consonants occur in English.

The complete analysis of data is represented schematically in Table 4. A more detailed discussion of the analysis of the individual error types will be found in subsequent chapters.

TABLE 4

Analysis of Data

<table>
<tr><td colspan="12">Error Types</td></tr>
<tr><td colspan="3">phoneme substitution</td><td colspan="2">simplification</td><td colspan="2">addition</td><td colspan="5">environment</td></tr>
<tr><td>1 distinctive feature</td><td colspan="2">1+ distinctive feature</td><td rowspan="2">syllable</td><td rowspan="2">phoneme</td><td rowspan="2">syllable</td><td rowspan="2">phoneme</td><td colspan="2">intra-morphemic blends</td><td colspan="2">inter-morphemic blends</td><td rowspan="2">metathesis</td></tr>
<tr><td>markedness</td><td>2 distinctive features</td><td>2+ distinctive features</td><td>P</td><td>R</td><td>P</td><td>R</td></tr>
<tr><td colspan="12">phonological context</td></tr>
</table>

3

BASES FOR ANALYSIS

In the linguistic investigation of normal speech, certain assumptions are made about the linguistic competence and performance of the speaker. It is tacitly assumed that all normal adults have complete command of the phonological system of the language including the complete repertory of phonemes with their rules of occurrence and combination, and that each speaker reflects this competence in verbal output. With these assumptions firmly established, the investigator proceeds to analyze his data linguistically.

In investigating pathological speech, however, no such assumptions can be made. There is no a priori reason to expect that the phonological patterns of aphasic speech will follow the phonological distributions and constraints found in normals. For example, it is conceivable that the aphasic has an incomplete phonemic inventory and that certain phonemes or classes of phonemes are eliminated from his verbal output. Therefore, to begin a linguistic analysis of the phonological errors made by aphasics, without determining the distribution of the features in their total speech pattern, is premature. Rather, it is necessary to determine the distributional patterns which are representative of aphasic speech and compare these results to normal frequency distributions. Only after a norm is established can the analysis of phonological errors be undertaken.

An analysis of frequency distributions is important for more than the methodological reasons discussed above. It has been observed in areas of developmental and pathological psycholinguistics that frequency of occurrence of words or utterances has a direct effect on the availability and correct usage of the item in the speech repertory. For example, it has been noted that the verbal output of aphasics is characterized by an overuse of high frequency words and dearth of low frequency words.[1] Moreover, the frequency of an item seems to be correlated with its correct use, i.e. the higher its frequency, the lower the chance of errors. If frequency plays such a fundamental role in speech behavior on the word or utterance level, it is conceivable that this factor would also be reflected in the distribution of phonemic errors in aphasic speech. Thus, it would be expected that the frequency of an error made on a specific phoneme would be inversely correlated with its frequency of occurrence; the most common phonemes will have proportionately fewer errors than the least common phonemes of the inventory.

It is the object of this chapter to establish the bases pre-requisite to a linguistic analysis of aphasic speech. Several analyses were made to achieve this end: (I) the phonological patterns representative of aphasic speech were determined and compared to normal frequency distributions; (II) The distribution of phonemic errors was studied in relation to the distribution of target phonemes in aphasic speech.

ANALYSIS I: Phoneme Frequency Distributions

The sample for this analysis consisted of two aphasics chosen randomly from each diagnostic group – Broca's, Conduction, and Wernicke's. The spontaneous speech of each patient was transcribed using the International Phonetic Alphabet until 1000 consonant phonemes were obtained. The frequencies tabulated were based on the actual phonemes produced by the aphasic patients and not on

[1] c.f. J. Wepman, R. Bock, L. Jones, D. van Pelt, "Psycholinguistic study of aphasia: a revision of the concept of anomia", *Journal of Speech and Hearing Disorders*, 21, 468–477 (1956); D. Howes and N. Geschwind, "Quantitative studies of aphasic language", in *Disorders of Communication*, ed. D. Rioch (Baltimore, 1964) 233; H. Goodglass, M. Hyde and S. Blumstein, "Frequency, picturability and availability of nouns in aphasia", *Cortex*, 5, 104–119 (1969) 108 ff.

the target phonemes. Moreover, dialectal variations and colloquial speech phenomena were not normalized.

The main distribution of phonemes was determined for the aphasic sample and compared to a normal distribution curve of English phonemes.[2] A Spearman Rank Order Correlation Coefficient Test was conducted to measure the degree of concordance between the consonant distributions reflected in aphasic and normal speech.

The similarity between the distributional patterns of the aphasics

TABLE 5

(%) *Consonant Phoneme Distributions in Normals and Aphasics*

	Normal	Aphasic
t	8.40	9.63
n	7.08	7.10
s	5.09	4.56
d	4.18	3.74
l	3.69	3.43
m	3.29	2.95
ð	2.99	3.06
k	2.90	2.69
r	2.77	4.41
w	2.57	2.86
z	2.49	2.32
b	2.08	2.26
v	1.85	1.50
p	1.77	1.01
f	1.72	1.67
h	1.67	1.25
y	1.53	1.72
ŋ	1.24	.63
g	1.16	1.53
š	.70	.39
θ	.60	.88
ǰ	.51	.40
č	.37	.19
ž	.05	.01

[2] P. B. Denes, "On the statistics of spoken English", *Journal of the Acoustical Society of America*, 35, 892–904 (1963) 894.

and normals is seen by inspection of the graph in Figure 2 and the mean percentage figures in Table 5. The rank order correlation was .95 ($p < .01$).

Thus, the phoneme distributions reflected in the spontaneous speech of aphasic patients does not seem to be different from that found in normal speech. This similarity of distribution is interesting in the light of obvious disturbances in phonology observed in aphasic speech. An analysis by phoneme distributions is not sensitive enough to differentiate pathological from normal speech.

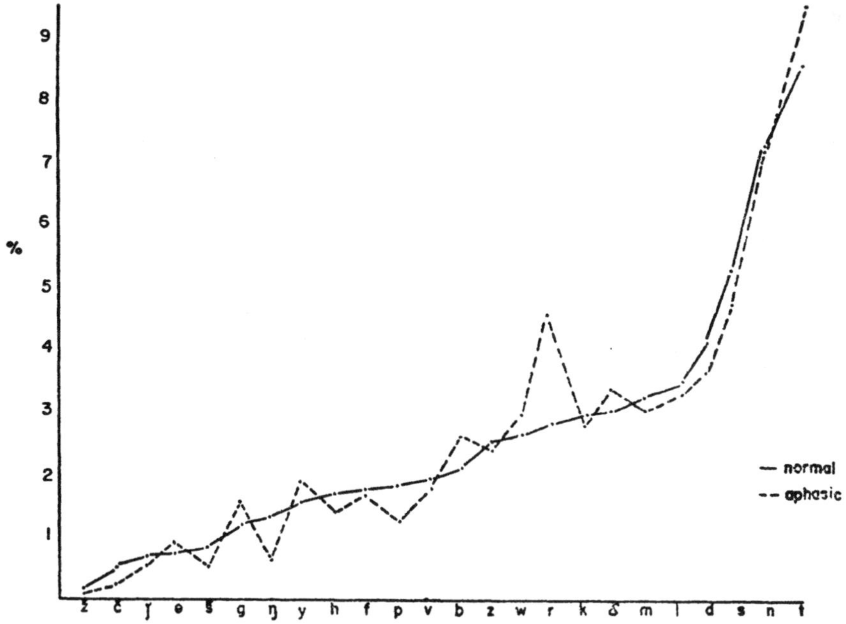

Fig. 2. Phoneme frequency distribution

ANALYSIS II: Distribution of Phoneme Errors

With the phonemic frequency distribution established for the aphasic sample, it is now possible to consider the relationship between phoneme error rate and frequency of occurrence. In order to measure this relationship, the ratio between the errors made on each phoneme and the actual frequency of occurrence of each phoneme in aphasic speech was computed $(\frac{\%\ \text{error}}{\%\ \text{occur.}})$. These results were graphed and compared to the rank order distribution of phonemes determined in Analysis I (see Figure 3).

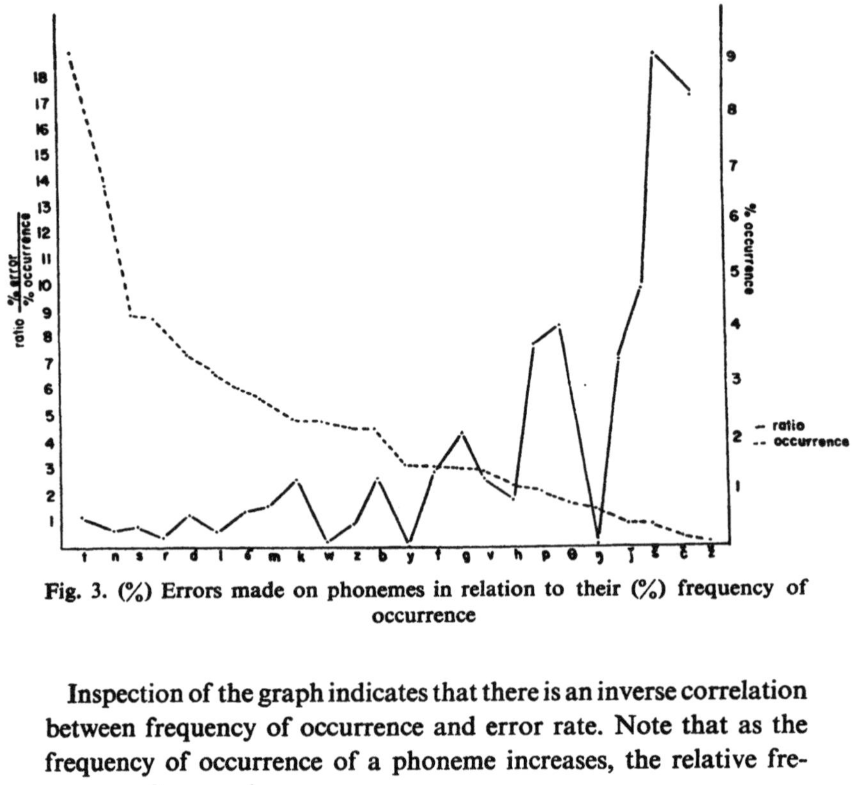

Fig. 3. (%) Errors made on phonemes in relation to their (%) frequency of occurrence

Inspection of the graph indicates that there is an inverse correlation between frequency of occurrence and error rate. Note that as the frequency of occurrence of a phoneme increases, the relative frequency of errors decreases.

Thus, it seems that frequency factors affect the aphasics' performance on the phonological level as well as other linguistic levels. The inverse correlation between frequency of occurrence and error rate suggests that there may be some characteristics intrinsic to the phonemic code which make some sounds inherently more difficult or complicated to produce than others. An analysis of the 'behavior' of the phonemes in aphasic speech – i.e. the types and directions of errors made – may give some insights into the organization of the phonological system as well as the relationships between the phonemes comprising the system. Only after this is understood can the factors contributing to the ease or difficulty of production be determined.

4

DISTINCTIVE FEATURE AND MARKEDNESS ANALYSIS

4.1. DISTRIBUTION OF ERROR TYPES

The phonological errors characteristic of aphasic speech include errors of phoneme substitution, simplification, addition, and environmental influence. In order to determine if these error types reflected a given order of difficulty in the aphasic sample, the distribution of errors made within each group was examined.

The mean percent of each error type was determined for each aphasic group. The distribution of errors made was ranked for each group and the probability of occurrence for this distribution was computed.

The distribution of errors based on raw scores of 1993, 590, and 219 errors for Broca's, Conduction, and Wernicke's aphasics respectively is seen in Table 6 and Figure 4. The rank order correlation coefficient for the aphasic sample is 1.0; i.e. each group had the same order of phonological errors made ($p < .01$).

These results support the original hypothesis; namely, that the

TABLE 6

Distribution of Aphasic Errors

	Broca	Conduction	Wernicke
phoneme substitution	48.7 %	52.7 %	35.2 %
simplification	24.7 %	24.3 %	30.3 %
environment	20.0 %	15.4 %	20.7 %
addition	6.6 %	7.6 %	13.8 %

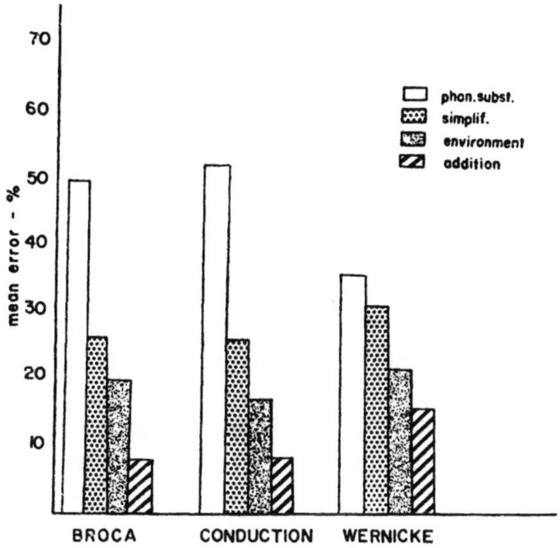

Fig. 4. Distribution of aphasic errors

types of errors made follow the same order of impairment in each aphasic group. It would seem then that the phonological errors characteristic of aphasic speech reflect a systematic disorganization of phonology independent of a particular lesion site.

It is necessary to emphasize, however, that the results obtained and the conclusions drawn can not be separated from the total configuration of the aphasic's behavior without obscuring some real differences which do, in fact, exist among the three aphasic groups considered. A look at the raw scores will demonstrate this quite clearly. As indicated above, the total number of errors made by each group are:

Broca	Conduction	Wernicke
1993	590	219

The range in errors made reflects a factor commonly observed in clinical testing – Broca's aphasics seem to have considerably more trouble with the phonological system than fluent aphasics (Conduction and Wernicke's) and within the fluent group, Conduction aphasics seem to be more impaired than Wernicke's.

4.2. PHONEME SUBSTITUTIONS: ERRORS OF ONE DISTINCTIVE FEATURE

The error type most seriously affected in all aphasic groups was the category phoneme substitution (see Table 6). It is the object of the rest of this chapter to investigate the concept distinctive feature with relation to this class of error and to test the applicability of the distinctive feature framework as hypothesized by Jakobson, Halle, and Fant to an analysis of aphasic speech. The first analysis tests the assumption that phoneme substitution errors are more likely to occur between phonemes related by single feature differences than between phonemes related by multiple feature differences.

To this end, phoneme substitution errors were classified into errors of one or more than one distinctive feature. The mean percent for each classification was determined for each aphasic group. The distribution of errors was tested for deviation from the natural chance distribution by means of a two-tailed binomial approximation test with Yate's correction. The percents computed are based on raw scores of 1003, 311, and 79 for Broca's, Conduction, and Wernicke's respectively.

The distribution of distinctive feature errors within each aphasic group was significant beyond the .01 level: Broca's = 13.07, Conduction = 10.73, and Wernicke's = 4.85. A graph comparing these distributions is found in Figure 5. The similarity of the distinctive feature errors across groups is striking. Note that the difference across groups of errors of one and more than one distinctive feature is less than 5 %.

Two fundamental conclusions can be drawn from these results. Firstly, the hypothesis that distinctive feature errors are more likely to occur between phonemes related by a single feature than phonemes separated by several features is strongly supported. Secondly, the

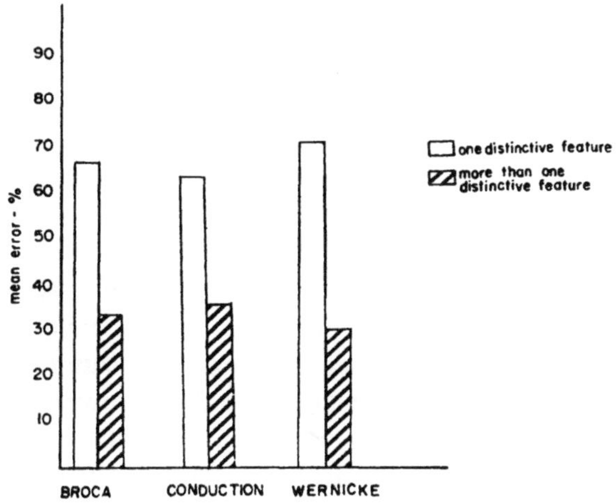

Fig. 5. Phoneme substitutions: Distinctive feature analysis

similar distributions of one and more than one distinctive feature errors across groups further substantiates the hypothesis that the same patterns of phonological dissolution will be found throughout the aphasic sample.

4.3 HIERARCHY OF FEATURES

The one distinctive feature errors were then analyzed to test the assumption that the features characterizing the phonological system are differently but systematically affected in aphasic speech, and moreover, that the errors reflect the hierarchical organization of features hypothesized by Roman Jakobson.

This hierarchy was proposed by Jakobson in his discussion of phonemic patterning in language acquisition.[1] According to him, the order of consonant features acquired is:

[1] Jakobson and Halle, *Fundamentals*, A1.

consonant
{ nasal
grave }[2]
{ compact
voice }
continuant
strident

Since this hierarchy implies a given order of difficulty, it would be expected that the patterns of feature disintegration in aphasic speech would be the inverse of the patterns of feature acquisition – i.e. more aphasic errors would occur in those features acquired last and fewer errors in those features acquired first.

To test this hypothesis, each one distinctive feature error was classified according to the distinctive feature modified; i.e. compact, grave, nasal, voice, strident, and continuant. The mean percent of errors made on each feature was calculated for each aphasic group. These results were then arranged in descending order of frequency and compared (see Table 7).

TABLE 7

Hierarchy of Feature Dissolution

Broca		Conduction		Wernicke	
continuant	39.0 %	continuant	26.2 %	compact	41.6 %
compact	19.8 %	compact	25.4 %	continuant	16.8 %
voice	16.6 %	grave	20.4 %	voice	16.6 %
grave	10.8 %	voice	15.3 %	grave	12.5 %
nasal	9.3 %	strident	7.3 %	strident	10.5 %
strident	4.5 %	nasal	5.4 %	nasal	2.0 %

It can be immediately seen that the hierarchical organization of errors is not the same for each group and that the percent of errors made on each feature varies considerably. Rank order correlations conducted between each group – Broca-Conduction, Conduction-

[2] The brackets {} indicate that the order of the features is not strictly defined.

Wernicke, and Broca-Wernicke were not significant ($r^s = .542$ for each correlation).

Although the distribution of errors is not the same in each group, there does seem to be a general pattern underlying the hierarchies established. Note in the Table that the feature hierarchy seems to be divided into triads; i.e. the two most common feature errors made within each aphasic group are either [continuant] or [compact]; the next most frequent errors are either [grave] or [voice]; and finally, the fewest errors are made with the features [strident] or [nasal]. Thus, within the specific limits established by the triad, the feature arrangement does seem to be consistent and systematic.

On the whole, there seems to be a relationship between the hypothesized hierarchy and the organization of features demonstrated by the aphasic data. Compare:

ACQUISITION	APHASIC DATA
consonant	consonant
{ nasal, grave }	{ nasal, strident }
{ compact, voice }	{ grave, voice }
continuant	{ compact, continuant }
strident	

Note that except for the feature [strident], the feature hierarchy for the aphasics is consistent with the feature hierarchy suggested by Jakobson.

There are two factors which may have contributed to the relative sparseness of strident errors observed in the aphasic data. Firstly, unlike the other distinctive features, [strident] has a very limited distribution, i.e. it is used only to differentiate two groups of phonemes – $\left[\begin{smallmatrix}\check{c}\\ \check{j}\end{smallmatrix}\right]$ – $\left[\begin{smallmatrix}k\\ g\end{smallmatrix}\right]$ and $\left[\begin{smallmatrix}s\\ z\end{smallmatrix}\right]$ – $\left[\begin{smallmatrix}\theta\\ \eth\end{smallmatrix}\right]$. All of the other features distinguish a larger number of phoneme classes, and consequently, by frequency factors alone, the possibility for errors is sharply increased. In this sense, then, strident is a 'defective' feature.

Secondly, the frequency of the phonemes $\left\{\begin{smallmatrix}\check{c}\\ \check{j}\end{smallmatrix}\right\}$ is very limited in

English. It will be remembered that in the analysis conducted in Chapter 3 considering the percent of errors on individual phonemes in relation to their frequency of occurrence, a proportionately large number of errors occurred with low frequency phonemes as $\left\{\begin{smallmatrix}\check{c}\\ \check{j}\end{smallmatrix}\right\}$ (see Figure 3). Thus, if the proportion of feature changes were considered in relation to the frequency of occurrence of the phonemes $\left\{\begin{smallmatrix}\check{c}\\ \check{j}\end{smallmatrix}\right\}$, the percent of stridency errors would have a higher incidence than was demonstrated in the analysis of features, based solely on absolute occurrences of errors.

4.4. PHONEME SUBSTITUTION ERRORS : MARKEDNESS ANALYSIS

Based on the assumption that the values of the features characterizing the phonemes of the system are hierarchically organized, it was hypothesized that in the dissolution of aphasic speech, the marked structures would be impaired in relation to the relative preservation of the more basic or unmarked structures. Thus, it would be expected that most phoneme substitution errors will involve the substitution of an unmarked for a marked phoneme.

To test this assumption, each phoneme substitution error characterized by a single feature change was classified according to the direction of the error made; either the phoneme change was from a marked consonant to an unmarked consonant, e.g. *n* → *d*, or the change was from an unmarked to a marked consonant, e.g. *d* → *n*. The mean percent of errors in each category was calculated for each aphasic group. These percents were based on raw scores of 645 for Broca's, 182 for Conduction, and 57 for Wernicke's aphasics.[3]

The distribution of errors was tested for deviation from the

[3] It may be noted that these scores are smaller than the total number of phoneme substitution errors of one distinctive feature discussed in Section 4.2 (Broca's 681, Conduction 199, Wernicke's 58). The exact markedness relations between the phoneme pairs $\left[\begin{smallmatrix}p-t\\ b-d\end{smallmatrix}\right]$ is one of the questions still being discussed in current linguistic theory. Consequently, these error types were separated from the main body of data and are considered in Chapter 8.

natural chance distribution by means of a two-tailed binomial approximation test with Yate's correction. Results were significant for Broca's and Wernicke's aphasics (Broca's : $z = 7.5_{p < .01}$; Wernicke's : $z = 9.46_{p < 0.1}$) but non-significant for the Conduction group (Conduction: $z = 1.11$). A graph comparing these distributions is found in Figure 6. Note the striking similarity be-

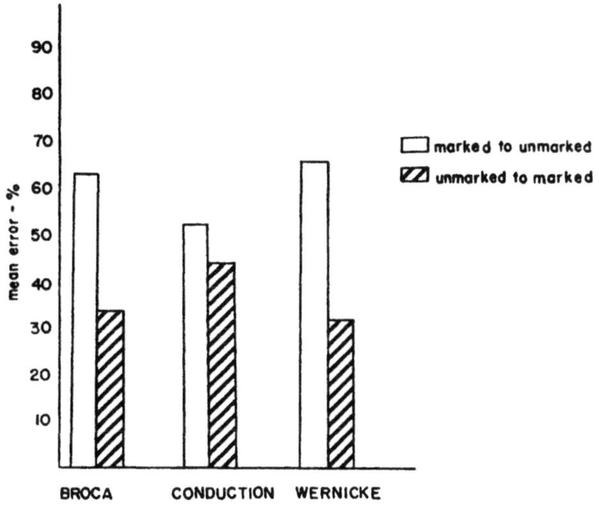

Fig. 6. Markedness analysis

tween the distribution of markedness errors in the Broca's and Wernicke's aphasics – the error distributions differed by less than 3 %.

Despite the fact that the Conduction aphasics' error distributions are non-significant, the direction of errors made does reflect a tendency for marked consonants to become unmarked. In view of this tendency and of the significant results shown by the other two groups, it can be inferred that the data support the hypothesis that unmarked consonants will tend to be substituted for marked consonants more often than the reverse.

5

CONTEXTUAL ANALYSIS OF PHONOLOGICAL ERRORS

The previous chapter has established that the phonological disintegration of aphasic speech can be systematically described. The analyses made were concerned specifically with the types of phonological errors comprising the phonological patterns of aphasic speech, and subsequently, with the characterization of the class of phoneme substitution errors by use of the notions distinctive feature and markedness. In these analyses, no attempt was made to determine the relationship, if any, between the errors made and the phonological context in which the errors occurred. Thus, for example, all phoneme substitution errors were analyzed together regardless of whether an error occurred in initial position or embedded within a cluster in word medial position. It is the object of this chapter to investigate the contexts of the phonological errors made to determine: (1) if, in general, phonological errors are restricted to specific contexts; (2) if there are consistent differences in the contexts in which the four error categories – phoneme substitution, simplification, addition, and environment – are found.

5.1. CONTEXTUAL ANALYSIS OF PHONEME SUBSTITUTION ERRORS

The first area of investigation was concerned with phoneme substitution errors.[1] Each error was assigned to a category defined by the context in which it occurred. These categories included:

CONTEXT	EXAMPLE (ITALIC LETTER)
$\# -$	'*c*at'
$\# - C$	'*s*ting'
$\# C -$ (r,l,w)	'p*l*ate'
$\# C -$	's*t*ing'
$\# CC -$	'st*r*ing'
$\# - CC$	'*s*tring'
$\# C - C$	's*t*ring'
$V - V$	'ba*b*y'
$XC - X$	'cus*t*omer'
$X - CX$	'cu*s*tomer'
$XCC - X$	'administ*r*ation'
$X - CCX$	'admini*s*tration'
$XC - CX$	'adminis*t*ration'
$- \#$	'pi*n*'
$C - \#$	'pin*t*'
$- C \#$	'pi*n*t'
$CC - \#$	'pint*s*'
$- CC \#$	'pi*n*ts'
$C - C \#$	'pin*t*s'

where $\#$ = word boundary, $\# -$ = word initial position and $- \#$ word final position; $X - X$ = within a word; C = consonant, V = vowel.

Because the percentage scores for cluster errors were so small for each group, the results were combined under three major headings: $\underline{\# -}$ * comprising all clusters in initial position ($\# - C$, $\# - CC$, $\# C -$ where $-$ = r,l,w, $\# C -$, $\# C - C$), $\underline{X - X}$ comprising all clusters in medial position ($XC - X$, $XCC - X$, $XC - CX$, $X - CX$),

[1] A preliminary analysis of the contextual distribution of one distinctive feature and more than one distinctive feature phoneme substitution errors was very similar. Consequently, the groups were combined and will be considered here as a single category. For a detailed discussion see S. Blumstein, *Phonological Implications of Aphasic Speech*, doctoral dissertation, Harvard University (1970).

and – # * comprising all clusters in final position (*C* – #, *CC* – #, – *C* #, – *CC*#, *C* – *C* #, *CC* – #).

The results of the analysis, based on raw scores of 897, 271, and 72, for Broca's, Conduction, and Wernicke's aphasics respectively, are seen in Table 8. Except for Wernicke's aphasics, most phoneme

TABLE 8

Phoneme Substitution Errors: Contextual Distribution

	Broca	Conduction	Wernicke
#–	53.6 %	45.9 %	27.7 %
V–V	14.5 %	17.8 %	19.6 %
–#	9.7 %	13.4 %	29.3 %
#–*	11.7 %	7.1 %	5.6 %
X–X	7.7 %	12.1 %	11.8 %
–#*	2.8 %	3.7 %	6.0 %

substitution errors occurred when the target phoneme was in word initial position.

Clearly, in all groups, most substitution errors occurred with single consonants, i.e. initially, medially, or finally. Compare:

Phoneme Substitution Errors

	Broca	Conduction	Wernicke
single *C*	77.7 %	77.1 %	76.7 %
cluster	22.3 %	22.9 %	23.3 %

It is clear that the position of a phoneme in a word does affect the frequency with which an error is made. The fact that most errors occur in word initial position suggests that the patterns observed may be conditioned by frequency factors based on English word structure. Since most words in English begin with a single consonant, it follows that there are more opportunities for errors to occur in this context. If frequency factors alone are responsible for the patterns observed, there should be a positive correlation between the number of errors made in a specific context and the frequency of occurrence of that particular context in English word structure. An analysis was conducted to test this hypothesis.

Transcribed samples of interviews with Broca's and Wernicke's aphasics were used in this analysis. The consonants used in 2000 consecutive words were categorized according to their contextual positions. Since the word choice of aphasics might be sufficiently different from normal to affect the general distribution of phonological contexts, a comparable sample was analyzed of normal speech. The mean percent occurrence for each contextual category was computed for each group. The results were graphed and compared to the contextual distribution of phoneme substitution errors in Broca's and Wernicke's aphasics (see Figure 7).

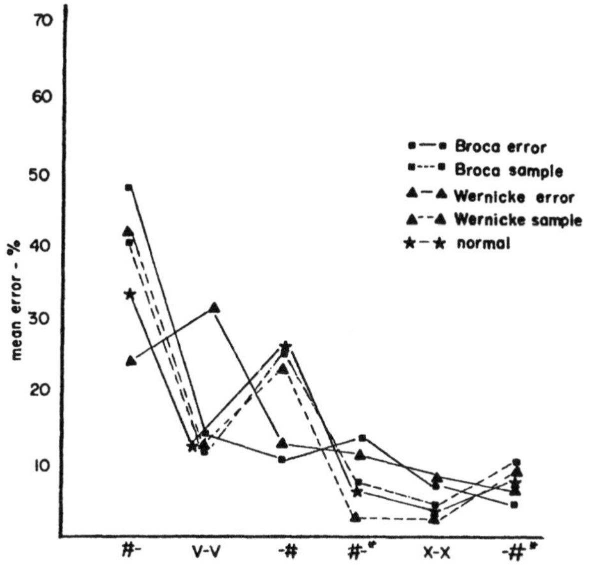

Fig. 7. Distribution of environments of consonant phonemes

A comparison of the contextual distributions in the aphasic and normal sample reveals no apparent differences – the shape of the distribution curves are the same and the frequency of errors in each category is strikingly similar. Thus, the word structure of normals and aphasics is considered comparable.

A comparison of the distribution of phonological contexts found in the analysis of substitution errors, on the one hand, and the analysis of word structure, on the other, indicates a positive correlation in all groups between frequency of occurrence and errors in clusters within a word ($X - X$) and in word final positions ($- \# *$). However, although the errors follow frequency distributions in word initial position ($\# -$) and in word medial position ($V - V$) for Broca's aphasics, they do not coincide for the Wernicke's aphasics. Moreover, for both groups the distribution of errors in word final position ($- \#$) and in initial cluster position ($\# - *$) does not coincide with the frequency of occurrence of consonant phonemes in this environment.

On the basis of this analysis, it is concluded that frequency factors alone cannot account for the distribution of phoneme substitution errors made. Another possible explanation is suggested by the distributional patterns of substitution errors observed. The most consistent finding in the substitution analysis was the over-riding abundance in all groups of errors in the context of single consonants. It is suggested that the tendency for errors to occur in the context of single consonants versus clusters is a direct function of the underlying differences involved in coding and programming for production single consonants, on the one hand, and consonant clusters, on the other.

The production of sequences of consonants and vowels does not simply involve the juxtaposition of discrete phonemic entities. Instead, the successive sounds of speech exert a considerable influence on each other. For example, the production of /k/ in the words 'key' and 'cool' varies due to the anticipation of the front vowel /i/ or the back vowel /u/.

Thus, the articulatory program necessary for the production of syllabic sequences demands a complex integration of articulatory movements. As the syllabic structure becomes more complex, the sequential dependencies necessary for proper coding and production increase. In this way, the segments comprising the structure are more strictly bound to the unit as a whole, and, in this sense, have less structural independence. It is the nature of this complex bond which seems to inhibit substitution errors within consonant clusters.

The nature of the syllable structure in *CV* sequences, however, is less complex. Because the domain in which the individual segments are contained is much smaller, the phonological constraints are less. Consequently, each segment is less intrinsically bound to the unit and, as a result, substitution errors can occur without severely disrupting programmed syllable structures.

5.2. ANALYSIS OF SIMPLIFICATION AND ADDITION ERRORS

Unlike substitution errors, errors of simplification and addition change the syllable structure of the target word attempted. Thus, a consonant is either dropped from or added to a specific phonological environment. It is the object of this section to analyze the simplification and addition errors made by aphasics and then consider these results in relation to those obtained in the previous section.

As indicated in Chapter 4, the distribution of simplification errors in the aphasic sample was 24.7 %, 24.3 %, and 30.3 % for Broca's ,Conduction, and Wernicke's aphasics respectively. Two types of simplification errors were made. In the first, an entire syllable was lost, e.g. /viEtnamiz/ 'Vietnamese' → /biEtmiz/. In the second, a single consonant was lost, e.g. /ski/ 'ski' → /si/. The contextual analysis of simplification errors will be limited to the second category.

As in the previous section, the consonant simplification errors

TABLE 9

Consonant Simplification Errors: Contextual Distribution

	Broca	Conduction	Wernicke
#—	9.9 %	9.4 %	1.2 %
V—V	1.3 %	.5 %	—
—#	15.5 %	16.6 %	14.7 %
#—*	29.7 %	22.2 %	28.8 %
X—X	18.8 %	20.2 %	28.2 %
—#*	24.8 %	31.1 %	27.1 %

were classified into the following categories: $\# -$, $V - V$, $- \#$, $\# - *$, $X - X$, $- \# *$. The mean percent of errors made in each category was computed for each aphasic group.

The results of this analysis, based on raw scores of 391, 109, and 48 errors for Broca's, Conduction, and Wernicke's aphasics respectively are seen in Table 9.

Note that the large majority of simplification errors occurred in the context of consonant clusters:

	Broca	Conduction	Wernicke
single *C*	26.7 %	26.5 %	15.9 %
cluster	73.3 %	73:5 %	84.1 %

Moreover, the simplification of these clusters is distributed fairly evenly in initial, medial and final position. This distribution suggests that the errors made are conditioned by the complexity of the syllable structure rather than by the position of the cluster in the word. Of the simplification errors made in the environment of single consonants, most errors for all groups occurred in word final position.

The distribution of simplification errors demonstrates the wide applicability and importance of the notion markedness in phonology. Phonological theory hypothesizes that the basic, canonical, or unmarked form of a syllable is universally *CV*. Other syllabic structures as *CCV* which have smaller distributional domains, are learned later by the child, and are phonologically more complex, are marked.

The pattern of simplification errors clearly demonstrates the tendency for marked syllable structures to become unmarked. On the one hand, consonant clusters are simplified, thus reducing the complexity of the syllable structure; on the other, when a single consonant is lost, it tends to be lost in final position, thus reducing the syllable structure from *CVC* to *CV*, the unmarked form.

The addition errors made by the aphasics constituted the smallest category of errors made – 6.6 % for Broca's ,7.6 % for Conduction, and 13.8 % for Wernicke's. There were two types of addition errors – the addition of a syllable to a target word, e.g. /klawdi/ 'cloudy' → /kəlawdi/, and the addition of a consonant to a target word, e.g. /Eləvetɔr/ 'elevator' → /kEləvetɔr/. As in the case of the simplification errors, the analysis of the contexts in which errors occurred will be limited to consonant additions.

The addition errors made were grouped into the following categories: # –, – #, # – *, X – X, – # *.[2] The mean percent of errors made in each category was determined for each aphasic group. The percentage scores found in Table 10 are based on a total of 111 errors for Broca's ,40 for Conduction, and 22 for Wernicke's aphasics.

TABLE 10

Consonant Addition Errors: Contextual Distribution

	Broca	Conduction	Wernicke
#–	26.0 %	28.5 %	30.6 %
–#	10.2 %	11.5 %	13.5 %
#–*	28.5 %	38.5 %	30.2 %
X–X	33.0 %	12.9 %	11.9 %
–#*	2.3 %	8.6 %	13.8 %

It is obvious from the distribution of contexts in which addition errors took place that most errors occurred in consonant clusters, thus complicating further the syllable structure of the target word. Hence,

	Broca	Conduction	Wernicke
single C	37.2 %	40.0 %	43.1 %
clusters	62.8 %	60.0 %	56.9 %

In considering these errors, it was noted that consonants were not

[2] Note that the category V – V is not included in this list. In English, vowels functioning as syllabic peaks are not juxtaposed without an intervening consonant, and consequently, there were no possibilities for errors to occur in this environment.

randomly added to the several contexts analyzed, but rather, the specific errors made were often motivated by the surrounding phonological context. Of all addition errors made, only three types constantly recurred: (1) $V \rightarrow \# CV$: This type involves the addition of a consonant before an initial vowel, e.g. /armi/ 'army' → /ǰarmi/. This is the only environment in which the addition of a consonant theoretically simplifies syllable structure. Here, the marked syllable structure ($\# V$) becomes the basic, canonical, and thus unmarked form ($\# CV$); (2) ARTICULATORILY BASED: The consonant added to a syllable was similar in place but different in manner to the consonant in the target syllable, e.g. /sawθ/ 'south' → /stawθ/, /wEpənz/ 'weapons' → /wEpmənz/; and (3) $C \rightarrow C \left\{ \begin{smallmatrix} \text{liquid} \\ \text{semi-}C \end{smallmatrix} \right\}$: This error type involved the addition of a liquid or semi-consonant to a stop or continuant, thus producing the most common consonant clusters in English, e.g. /tami/ 'Tommy' → /trami/, /beisbɔl/ 'baseball' → /beisbrɔl/.

The frequency with which these errors occur is seen below:

	Broca	Conduction	Wernicke
$\# V \rightarrow \# CV$	24.5 %	27.7 %	30.6 %
artic. based	23.5 %	9.7 %	19.5 %
$C \rightarrow C \left\{ \begin{smallmatrix} \text{liquid} \\ \text{semi-}C \end{smallmatrix} \right\}$	26.9 %	27.1 %	10.7 %
other	25.1 %	35.5 %	39.2 %

Between 60 % and 75 % of all addition errors can be motivated by the phonological context. Consequently, although additions may complicate the phonological structure, in general, they are motivated by the particular context in which they occur.

5.3 ENVIRONMENT ERRORS

Another set of errors clearly directed by their relationship to the syntagma are the environment errors. Included in this category are intra-morphemic blends, inter-morphemic blends, and metatheses. As defined in Chapter 2, intra-morphemic blends are characterized by a phoneme substitution error triggered by a phoneme located in the same word, e.g. 'Crete' → /trit/; inter-morphemic blends are assimilation errors triggered by phonemes located in neighboring words, e.g. 'roast beef' → /rof bif/; and metatheses are defined by the inversion of the order of phonemes in a given sequence, e.g. 'degrees' → /gədriz/.

In Chapter 4, the mean distribution of the category of environment errors was determined in relation to the other major types of phonological errors – phoneme substitution, simplification, and addition. These errors comprised 20.0 %, 15.4 %, and 20.7 % of the total in Broca's, Conduction, and Wernicke's groups respectively. The distribution of the types of environmental errors made by each aphasic group can be seen below:

	Broca	Conduction	Wernicke
intra-morphemic blends	52.6 %	44.3 %	31.5 %
inter-morphemic blends	26.8 %	36.3 %	56.7 %
metatheses	20.6 %	19.4 %	11.8 %

In order to ascertain the nature of each of these categories, a series of analyses was undertaken. The first was concerned with the distribution of progressive and regressive assimilations in intra-morphemic and inter-morphemic blends, and the second set was concerned with the relationship between the individual error categories (inter-, intra-morphemic blends, and metathesis) and the contexts in which these errors occurred.

5.3.1. *Progressive-Regressive Assimilation Errors*

Inter-morphemic and intra-morphemic blend errors were categorized by the direction of the assimilation errors made: progressive assimilations, characterized by the assimilation of the target phoneme to a previously occurring phoneme, e.g. 'dog' → /dɔd/, and regressive assimilations, characterized by assimilations based on the anticipation of a phoneme later in the sequence, e.g. 'doll' →

/lal/. The mean percents of these categories was determined for each aphasic group.

The results are summarized in Table 11.

TABLE 11

Progressive-Regressive Assimilation Errors

		Broca	Conduction	Wernicke
intra-morphemic	R	73.5 %	67.2 %	56.2 %
blends	P	26.5 %	32.8 %	43.8 %
inter-morphemic	R	55.1 %	47.2 %	57.5 %
blends	P	44.9 %	52.8 %	42.5 %

Except for the intra-morphemic blends made by Conduction aphasics, the analyses show that more regressive assimilation errors occurred than progressive assimilation errors. The difference between these two categories is most clearly reflected in the intra-morphemic blend errors.

The occurrence of both progressive and regressive assimilation errors demonstrates that many of the error types found in aphasic speech do, in fact, reflect the natural linguistic processes common in all languages. That is to say, regressive and progressive assimilations, as well as metatheses, occur commonly in the historical phonology of all languages. In fact, it is interesting to note that the predominance of regressive over progressive assimilation errors in intra-morphemic blends parallels the greater frequency of assimilations in phonological change.

Besides their general applicability to linguistic processes, these results contribute to the understanding of the mechanisms necessary for speech production. The predilection for regressive assimilation errors suggests that the difficulty manifested by the error is related to the programming rather than the actual implementation of the utterance .In other words, the fact that a phoneme is replaced by one which occurs LATER in the syntagma indicates that the timing which determines the specific ordering of the utterance must be modified BEFORE the patterns of articulatory movements can be implemented. Once implemented, these patterns are organized into sequentially ordered articulatory movements. Thus, although it is possible for a produced articulatory movement to contaminate one which follows (by perseveration), it is impossible for it to affect one which has not yet occurred. These results lend further support to the assumption that the phonological patterns of aphasic speech reflect a disturbance of the phonological rather than simply the phonetic mechanisms of language.

5.3.2. *Contextual Analyses of Environment Errors*

An important factor in triggering assimilation errors (inter- and intra-morphemic blends) has been discussed by Jakobson. As he states, "The number of distinctive features in the phoneme (or the number of phonemes in a phonemic system) and the maximum number of phonemes in the word, as well as the number of their possibilities of distribution and the maximal number of phonemic distinctions within a word, increases by degrees in child language (or decreases by degrees in aphasia)".[3] Thus, in speech production, as well as comprehension, the greater the number of different features used in a given sequence, the more difficulty the subject has in either producing or perceiving the sequence in its entirety. For example, the sequence /baba/, /bama/ and /bana/ reflect a hierarchy of difficulty; in each example, the number of features distinguishing the consonants in the sequence increases: b-b are equal, b-m are distinguished by one feature – nasality, b-n are distinguished by two features – nasality and place. As a result, assimilation errors are more likely to occur in those sequences containing a greater number of contrasts, e.g. /bana/, than those containing fewer contrasts, e.g. /baba/ or /bama/. It is clear that these assimilation errors are triggered by syntagmatic factors.

These considerations add a new dimension to the study of phonological contexts in which errors occurred. However, because this chapter has dealt exclusively with the relationship between the phonological context or position of a consonant in a word and the

[3] *Child Language, Aphasia*, 85.

phonological errors made by aphasics, the analysis of assimilation errors will be restricted simply to the contexts in which these errors occurred.

An analysis of the environmental distribution of inter- and intra-morphemic blends reveals an interesting parallel with the environments of phoneme substitution errors. As with the phoneme substitution errors, the majority of intra- and inter-morphemic blend errors occurred in the environment of a single consonant, i.e. initially, medially, and finally.

Compare:

	Broca	Conduction	Wernicke
Intra-morphemic blends			
single *C*	60.4 %	78.8 %	79.2 %
cluster	39.6 %	21.2 %	20.8 %
Inter-morphemic blends			
single *C*	70.0 %	84.7 %	93.3 %
cluster	30.0 %	15.3 %	6.7 %

Here again, the occurrence of a phonological error seems to be directly related to the complexity of the syllable structure. As syllabic complexity increases, sequential dependencies become greater, and each consonant which comprises the syllable seems in effect to have less structural independence .This seems to inhibit the occurrence of a phonological error. In contrast, in the production of a simpler syllabic structure as *CV*, the phonological constraints are less. Consequently, each segment is less intrinsically bound to the syllable structure and thus the possibility for errors seems to increase.

However, environmental errors are very different in nature from the other types of phonological errors made by aphasics. Unlike substitution, simplification, and addition errors, all elements motivating the occurrence of environmental errors exist in the target word or phrase – in the case of blend errors, it is the contaminating phoneme, and in the case of metathesis errors, it is the original order of phonemes. This suggests that it is not the bond between the particular error and its place of occurrence which is essential in characterizing the nature of environment errors, but rather the relationship between the phonological context of the particular error and the phonological context of the phoneme which triggers this error. This assumption was tested in each error category – intra-morphemic blends, e.g. 'good' → /dUd/; inter-morphemic blends, e.g. 'I think so' → /ai siŋk so/; and metathesis, e.g. 'elephant' → /Efələnt/.

The first error category to be considered was intra-morphemic blends. It was felt that the degree of relationship between a blend error and its contaminating phoneme was a function of the phonological distance between them; i.e. if, in general, a close bond existed between assimilated and contaminating phonemes in intra-morphemic blends, then regardless of the specific environment in which the error occurred, most errors would be triggered by phonemes in immediately contiguous contexts.

In order to test this assumption, the phonological distance measured by the number of consonant phonemes intervening between the blend error made and the contaminating phoneme in the target word was determined. This distance was measured by the following criteria: (1) if no consonants intervened between the assimilated phoneme and contaminating phoneme, it was categorized as a distance of 1, e.g. /big/ 'big' → /bi*b*/, /kIčən/ 'kitchen' → /kI*k*ən/; (2) if one consonant intervened, it was categorized as a distance of 2, e.g. /bIznəs/ 'business' → /bIz*b*əs/; (3) if two or more consonants intervened, it was categorized as a distance of 3, e.g. /spriŋtaim/ 'springtime' → /splI*n*saim/. The mean percent of errors in each category was determined for each aphasic group.

The results, based on raw scores of 210, 43, and 16 errors for Broca's, Conduction, and Wernicke's aphasics respectively, are summarized in Figure 8. It is clear that most assimilation errors occurred when the relationship between the triggering and assimilated phoneme was defined by the distance of 1. The disparity between the distribution of the distance 2 and 3 in Broca's and Conduction aphasics, on the one hand, and Wernicke's aphasics, on the other, could be due to the small number of errors com-

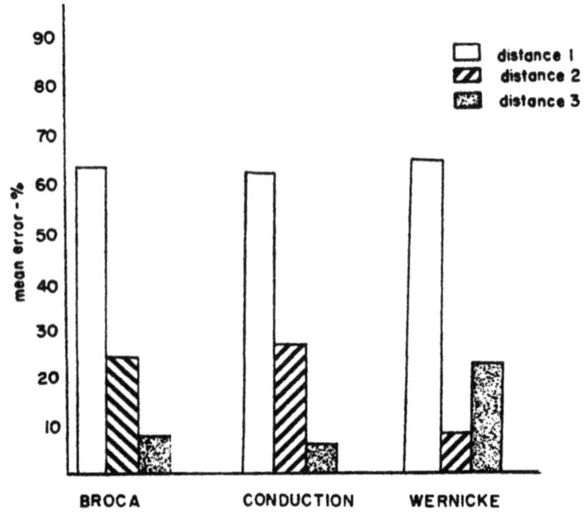

Fig. 8. Distance measure: intra-morphemic blends

prising the Wernicke's sample. Nevertheless, the relationship between the triggering phoneme and blend phoneme seems to be clearly characterized by the distance relation introduced above.

The notion of distance relation has wide applicability in all contextual errors. In the case of metatheses, this measure was used to determine the phonological distance a phoneme moved in the course of its transposition. Thus, if a consonant changed position either with the consonant nearest to it or with the vowel directly contiguous to it, it was categorized as a distance of 1, e.g. /mægəzin/ 'magazine' → /mæzəgin/, /kolts/ 'colts' → /klots/. If there was no reciprocal change in the position of the two consonants as above, but instead, one consonant was simply moved AROUND another, it was categorized as a distance of 2, e.g. /prəfEsər/ 'professor' → /pəfrEsər/. Any consonant which moved around two or more consonants was categorized as a distance of 3, e.g. /peistri/ 'pastry' → /preisti/.

The distance measure, based on the above criteria, was determined for each metathesis error made. The mean percent of error in each category was determined for the aphasic sample. The results, based on raw scores of 93 for Broca's, 21 for Conduction, and 9 for Wernicke's aphasics are seen in Figure 9. These results indicate that, in general, metathesis errors are characterized by the movement of a consonant within a strictly defined environmental framework.

The distance measure used above in the description of intra-morphemic blends and metathesis errors is not strictly applicable in the case of the final category – inter-morphemic blends. In the first two categories, the domain in which an error could occur was the word. However, inter-morphemic blends are defined by the assimilation of a phoneme in one word to another located in another word. It was realized that if the domain of the distance measure were extended across word boundaries, then the distance measure obtained would no longer characterize the relationship between the context of the contaminating and assimilated phoneme; instead, its value would increase or decrease as a function of the length of

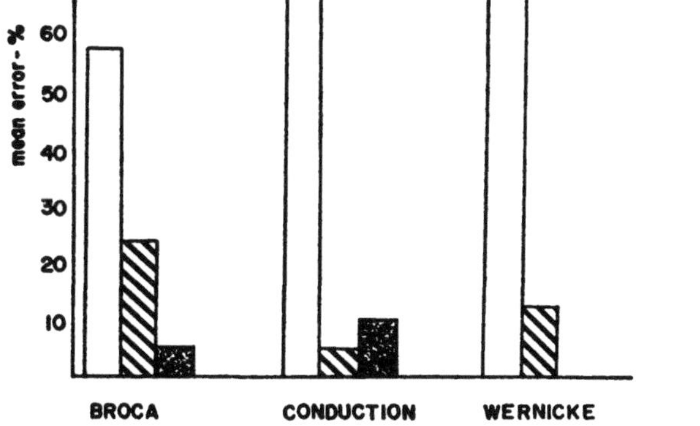

Fig. 9. Distance measure: metathesis

the word intervening between the assimilated and contaminating phoneme. This is clearly seen with the following examples:

(1) /ai hop so/ 'I hope so' → /ai sop so/
(2) /biutlfəl gr̩l/ 'beautiful girl' → /biutlfəl br̩l/

In the first example, the distance between the triggering phoneme and assimilated phoneme is one syllable. In the second, because the adjective is three syllables long, the distance measure is three syllables. Thus, this description fails to capture the fact that in both examples, the relationship between the contaminating and assimilated phoneme is the same, e.g. the phoneme assimilated is in the same structural environment as the contaminating phoneme.

It was this relationship which was thought to characterize the inter-morphemic blend errors. Consequently, an analysis based on a modified distance relation – the parallel structure relation – was made. This relation uses the parallel structure between the contaminating and assimilated phoneme as its basis of departure and then measures the phonological distance which the contaminating phoneme diverges from the structure of the assimilating phoneme. Thus, (1) if the assimilated phoneme was in the same context as the contaminating phoneme, then the error was categorized as a parallel structure relation. Differences in the syllable structure in which the contaminating and assimilated phoneme were located were not considered. In this way, parallel structure relations included errors of the type /hIstri bUks/ 'history books' → /bIstri bUks/ where the syllable structure in which the error occurred was the same as that of the assimilating phoneme – $\# CV$, as well as errors of the type /grin bəre/ 'green beret' → /brin bəre/ in which the initial consonant of the first word replaced the initial consonant of the second, although the syllable structure of the first was $\# C_1C_2V$ and that of the second was $\# CV$; (2) if the assimilated phoneme was in the same relative syllable but one consonant away from the parallel structure position of the contaminating phoneme, it was categorized as a distance of consonant 1, e.g. /no smok/ 'no smoke' → /no snok/; and (3) if the position of the assimilated phoneme was at least one syllable away from a parallel structure relation with the contaminating phoneme, it was categorized as a syllable 1 relation, e.g. /reiniŋ tudei/ 'raining today' → /reiniŋ turei/.

The mean percent of inter-morphemic blend errors made in each category was determined for each aphasic group. The results, based on raw scores of 210, 43, and 16 for Broca's, Conduction, and Wernicke's respectively, are found in Figure 10. Over 70 % of all

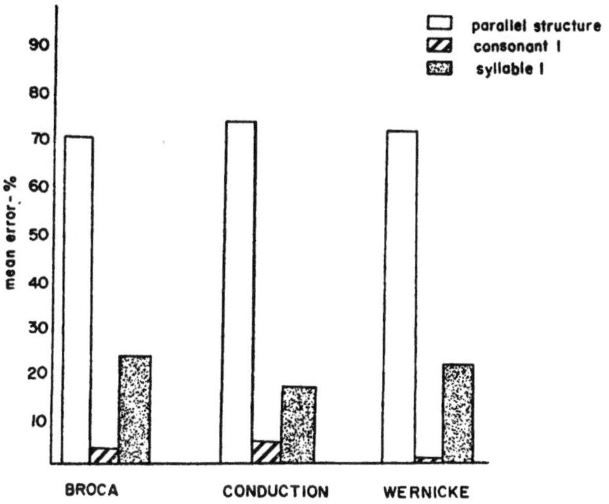

Fig. 10. Parallel structure measure: inter-morphemic blends

assimilation errors demonstrated a parallel structure relation to the contaminating phoneme. Moreover, most of the remaining errors that did not show the parallel structure relation were displaced to another syllable within the word rather than to a neighboring consonant.

In summary, the results of this chapter clearly demonstrate that each error type is intrinsically bound to the surrounding context. This relationship between paradigmatic and syntagmatic aspects of phonology forms a dynamic bond which characterizes the phonological pattern of aphasic speech. This is especially evident if all the error types and the various contexts in which they occurred are considered in relation to the phonological constraints of English. Out of 1993 errors for Broca's aphasics, 590 for Conduction, and

219 for Wernicke's, only 2.3 %, 3.3 % and 4.3 % for each group respectively were non-English sequences. In order for this to occur, the relationship between the type of error made and the context in which it occurred must form an integrated system, neither being able to function independent of the other.

Hence, although one distinctive feature phoneme substitution errors reflect the organization of the phonological system of English, their range of applicability is limited; for example, the phoneme substitution p → m never occurs in the environment # - l, # pl → *ml. Although theoretically any consonant can be assimilated to another following the parallel structure relation discussed above, its range of applicability is also limited. Thus, few assimilation errors result in a non-English sequence; for example, /rəniŋ hɔrs/ 'running horse' never becomes */rəniŋ hɔrsŋ/. This holds true for all types of phonological errors made.

In conclusion, the phonological system of the language cannot be properly understood without regard to both the paradigmatic and syntagmatic relations of phonology and the dynamic integration of the two.

6

IMPLICATIONS FOR APHASIA

The most consistent finding in the linguistic analysis of aphasic speech is the relative uniformity of error types and error directions in each aphasic group. The analysis of types of phonological errors, i.e. phoneme substitution, simplification, addition, and environment, revealed the same distributional pattern for each group; the distinctive feature analysis of phoneme substitution errors demonstrated that in all aphasic groups significantly more one distinctive feature errors were made than errors of more than one distinctive feature; a hierarchy of features was not only established for the aphasic sample as a whole but also closely paralleled the hierarchy proposed by Jakobson for the acquisition of language; the markedness analysis revealed a common tendency in all groups for unmarked values to be substituted for marked values; the analysis of the environments in which the types of phonological errors occurred demonstrated that each error type was directed by common principles – i.e. phoneme substitution and blend errors occurred predominantly in single consonant position; simplification errors reflected a tendency for marked syllable structures to become unmarked; addition errors were generally motivated by the phonological context in which they occurred; assimilation errors within a word and metathesis errors were conditioned by contiguous consonants; and blend errors across word boundaries reflected a similar structural relationship between the triggering and assimilated phoneme.

Thus, the phonological analysis of aphasic speech revealed no consistent differences among the three aphasic groups studied. And yet, clinically, these three aphasic groups are clearly distinguished. How, then, can these clinical differences be reconciled with the similar phonological patterns revealed in a linguistic analysis of aphasic speech?

Firstly, it is necessary to consider what the clinical examination purports to do. Essentially, it is a test designed to reveal a profile of language abilities and disabilities. Thus, the clinical examination is an investigation of language performance in all its modalities. It is the TOTALITY of the patient's performance on various linguistic tasks, and the relative impairment of one language modality over another which determines the patient's profile used in classifying the various aphasic syndromes. Although the clinical examination describes relative degree of impairment of various components or modalities of language, it does not attempt to determine the actual patterns of disintegration within a specific modality or linguistic task, nor is there any claim made about the similarities or differences of these patterns across groups. Thus, there is no contradiction in finding similar patterns of disintegration in phonology in the presence of three distinctly different clinical syndromes.

This can be seen most clearly with regard to the distinction made in the literature between phonetic disintegration characteristic of Broca's aphasics and phonemic disintegration characteristic of the posterior aphasics. The improper control of articulatory movements and the flattened intonational pattern often accompanying Broca's aphasia do indeed affect the total configuration and quality of speech production of the aphasic's performance. Thus, included in the speech pattern of these patients are phonological errors of the type defined here, i.e. errors involving distinctive values of the phonological system – phoneme substitution, simplification, addition, and environmental errors, as well as patterns of phonetic distortion superimposed on the patient's entire speech production. It is this dysarthric factor which dominates the clinical evaluation, and consequently, gives the impression that the quality of PHONOLOGICAL disintegration differs from the normally articulated but paraphasically produced speech characteristic of the syndrome phonemic disintegration. However, a systematic analysis of the

PHONOLOGICAL errors in all aphasic groups reveals similar patterns and distributions of errors. What qualitatively distinguishes these two syndromes then is not phonological disintegration characterized by the types of errors described in the literature and systematically analyzed here, but rather simply the presence or absence of a dysarthric quality of speech production.

It must be emphasized that the focus of this analysis has been concerned only with the verbal behavior of the speaker without including the problem of the factors triggering the production of phonological errors. The differences in quantity of error made by each aphasic group, on the one hand, and the different lesion sites producing three distinct profiles of language impairment, on the other, suggest that the mechanisms producing the phonological patterns under investigation may indeed be different in each aphasic group. However, despite any differences which may underlie the specific aphasic disorders, the patterns of phonological disintegration remain constant. This is the critical factor. For it suggests that the phonological system is hierarchically organized according to principles inherent to the language system, and it is this hierarchical organization of phonological relations which is reflected in the phonological patterns of aphasic speech.

Language then is seen as a highly integrated system organized according to a given set of hierarchically based universal rules or principles. It is always in relation to the system and its principles of organization that the phonological dissolution of speech can be characterized. Thus, regardless of the area of brain damage, the most complexly organized structures are impaired in contrast to the relative preservation of the less complex phonological structures.

PART II

IMPLICATIONS FOR PHONOLOGICAL THEORY

7

THE DISTINCTIVE FEATURE FRAMEWORK

In current phonological theory, the notion distinctive feature is of prime importance. Not only does it specify the individual components of which a phoneme is comprised but it also establishes the relationships among the phonemes of the phonological system of the language.

The phonological analysis of aphasic speech has supported many of the theoretical assumptions on which the notion distinctive feature is based. The analysis characterized the types of phoneme substitutions made by aphasics simply and insightfully and more importantly gave a principled explanation for the predilection of one type of phoneme substitution error over another; namely, that significantly more one distinctive feature errors were made by aphasics than errors of more than one distinctive feature, and the one distinctive feature substitution errors reflected a hierarchical disorganization of the features comprising the phonological system of English.

Further analysis of phoneme substitution errors, however, revealed some consistent discrepancies between the data and distinctive feature framework. Among the phoneme substitution errors of more than one distinctive feature, there was a constant recurrence of certain error types which theoretically should rarely, if ever, occur. Such frequent consonant confusions were:

$$\begin{Bmatrix} r \\ l \end{Bmatrix} \leftrightarrow w \qquad n \leftrightarrow l \qquad w \leftrightarrow m$$

$$\begin{Bmatrix} t \\ d \end{Bmatrix} \leftrightarrow l \qquad \begin{Bmatrix} v \\ b \end{Bmatrix} \leftrightarrow w \qquad \begin{Bmatrix} k \\ g \end{Bmatrix} \leftrightarrow h$$

The confusion of $\begin{Bmatrix} r \\ l \end{Bmatrix} \leftrightarrow w$, for example, necessitates a change in at least the features $\begin{bmatrix} \text{consonantal} \\ \text{vocalic} \end{bmatrix}$ –

$$\underset{\begin{bmatrix} + \text{ consonantal} \\ + \text{ vocalic} \end{bmatrix}}{r, l} \qquad\qquad \underset{\begin{bmatrix} - \text{ consonantal} \\ - \text{ vocalic} \end{bmatrix}}{w, y}$$

In fact, all of the above consonant confusions include a change in at least one or both of these features. An analysis of the aphasic data revealed that errors modifying class features as $\begin{bmatrix} \text{consonantal} \\ \text{vocalic} \end{bmatrix}$ occurred in all aphasic groups at least 2.5 times as often as phoneme substitution errors of 2 distinctive features e.g. $p \rightarrow v$, or more than two distinctive features, e.g. $p \rightarrow$ δ.[1]

According to the feature hierarchy established, these types of sound changes should occur infrequently. Moreover, according to the present theoretical framework, it would be just as likely for consonants $\begin{bmatrix} + \text{ consonantal} \\ - \text{ vocalic} \end{bmatrix}$ to be confused with vowels $\begin{bmatrix} - \text{ consonantal} \\ + \text{ vocalic} \end{bmatrix}$ as it is for liquids $\begin{bmatrix} + \text{ consonantal} \\ + \text{ vocalic} \end{bmatrix}$ to be confused with semi-consonants $\begin{bmatrix} - \text{ consonantal} \\ - \text{ vocalic} \end{bmatrix}$, a phenomenon which never occurs in aphasic speech. Thus, it would seem that the current distinctive feature framework does not adequately reflect all of the underlying phonemic relationships existing in the phonological system of the language.

Independent evidence from child language acquisition, historical linguistics, and dialectology also suggests that these phonemic relationships are not as uncommon as the present feature description would imply. Children not only commonly confuse liquids and semi-consonants, often after the rest of their phonemic inventory is acquired, but also have much difficulty distinguishing /v/ and /w/ in productive speech, e.g. 'the little boy' → [ðə wIɾl bɔi], 'Peter Rabbit' → [piɾr̥ wæbIt], 'very' → [wEri]. In historical phonology /k/ becomes /h/ in Old High German, e.g. makon → machōn 'make'. In certain dialectal forms of Latin, an alternation of /d/ and /l/ is

[1] For a detailed discussion of this analysis see Blumstein, *Phonological Implications*, 79 ff.

observed, e.g. *dingua* ~ *lingua* 'language', /w/ and /m/ alternate in dialects of Yokuts, an American Indian language, e.g. *imsa* ~ *iwsa* 'reciprocal morpheme' and /n/ and /l/ alternate in dialects of Taiwanese.[2]

All of the examples given above consist of changes involving liquids, semi-consonants, and nasals. It is just these classes of sounds which comprise the class sonorant described by Chomsky and Halle in *The Sound Pattern of English* (1968). They define sonorants as "sounds produced with a vocal tract cavity and configuration in which spontaneous voicing is possible".[3] The acoustic correlates seem to be the presence on the speech spectogram of periodic curves, rare presence of noise, and resonant bands.[4] Consequently, it would seem that the addition of the feature [sonorant] to the distinctive feature framework could characterize simply and insightfully the close relationship among liquids, glides, and nasals commonly found in linguistics proper as well as in aphasic speech.

The exact relationship between the feature [sonorant] and the distinctive feature framework proposed must now be considered. Its position in the hierarchy must be determined and its relation to the features used must be established. Moreover, its descriptive power must be tested, i.e. the feature [sonorant] must account only for those sounds intrinsically related. If it is too powerful, in the sense that it creates sound relations which, in fact, do not exist, then it is an inadequate construct and it must be subsequently modified.

The first area of investigation consists of those phonological

[2] I would like to thank Professors M. Silverstein and A. Arlotto for furnishing some of the examples used here.

[3] N. Chomsky and M. Halle, *The Sound Pattern of English* (New York, 1968) 302.

[4] c.f. T. Tarnóczy, "Resonance data concerning nasals, laterals and trills", in *Readings in Acoustic Phonetics*, ed. I. Lehiste (Cambridge, 1967) 111; L. Lisker, "Minimal cues for separating /w, r, l, y/ in intervocalic position", *Word*, 13, 256–267 (1957) 257; A. Liberman, "Some results of research in speech perception", reprinted in *Psycholinguistics*, ed. S. Saporta (New York, 1961) 146.

errors made within the sonorant class, i.e. $\text{sonorant}_1 \rightarrow \text{sonorant}_2$ where $1 \neq 2$, e.g. $r \rightarrow w$.

The most common errors made within this class are: $\begin{Bmatrix} r \\ l \end{Bmatrix} \leftrightarrow w$, $n \leftrightarrow l$, $w \leftrightarrow m$. The feature [compact] separates these phonemes from the remaining phonemes in the sonorant class; /w,r,l,m,n/ are [− compact] and /y,ŋ/ are [+ compact]. This group is further divided into two categories by the feature [nasal].

/w,r,l/	/m,n/
[− nasal]	[+ nasal]

Most phonological errors made within the sonorant class occurred between those sounds specified as $\begin{bmatrix} + \text{sonorant} \\ - \text{nasal} \\ - \text{compact} \end{bmatrix}$, i.e. /w,r,l/.

Further analysis of the data revealed many more errors between *w-r* than *w-l*. The distinctive feature framework should characterize this in some way. According to the distinctive feature framework of Jakobson, Halle, and Fant, /r/ and /l/ are differentiated in English by the feature [continuant], i.e. /r/ is [− continuant] and /l/ is [+ continuant]. /w/, on the other hand, is not specified for continuancy on the phonemic level. Thus, the feature [continuant] can not be used to characterize the relationship between /w/ and /r/. It would be possible to simply mark /w/ as [− continuant], thus relating it to /r/ and differentiating it from /l/. However, not only is continuancy a redundant feature for the semi-consonant /w/, but its introduction as a distinctive feature creates an ad hoc division on the phonemic level of the class of semi-consonants – i.e. /w/ would be specified and /y/ would be unspecified for continuancy on the phonemic level. To insure a uniform description of the class of semi-consonants, /y/ could also be marked for continuancy on the phonemic level, i.e. /y/ is [− continuant]. However, then the closer relationship between /w/ and /r/ versus /w/ and /l/ would not be expressed. On the basis of these factors, this analysis was considered inadequate.

In studying this problem, it seemed that the major difficulty in finding a solution was caused by the differentiation of /r/ and /l/ with the feature [continuant]. It is indeed questionable whether

/r/ in English is a non-continuant phoneme. Firstly, the articulation of /r/ is not characterized by an occlusion in the oral cavity followed by a sudden release. Rather, the tip of the tongue is curved upwards and retroflexed at the alveolar ridge while the air passes freely between the tongue tip and roof of the mouth. Moreover, the acoustic correlates of English /r/ are more similar to /l/ than to stop consonants. Non-continuants are characterized acoustically by a period of silence followed by a burst of noise at varying frequency levels. Both /r/ and /l/, on the other hand, are characterized acoustically by the presence of steady state resonance bands and are differentiated by a change in duration and relative intensity of these bands.[5] Hence, using the feature [continuant] to distinguish /r/ and /l/ does not seem motivated on the basis of either articulatory or acoustic criteria.

It is necessary to consider whether any other feature in the inventory could characterize the difference between /r/ and /l/. Of course, it is possible to simply introduce a new feature to account for these sounds. However, a decision to do this is a last measure since the use of a new feature must be motivated throughout the distinctive feature system established. Thus, it is preferable to find a solution within the existing framework.

A comparison of the articulation of /r/ and /l/ provides the clue to a possible analysis. As indicated earlier, /r/ is characterized by a retroflexion of the tongue tip toward the alveolar ridge. In addition, the sound is labialized, i.e. concomitant to the tongue position described, the lips are rounded. The tongue position for the articulation of /l/ is distinctly different; the tip of the tongue touches the alveolar ridge with the blade of the tongue extending back to the alveolar-palatal region. The air passes through laterally while the tongue is in this position. Moreover, no labialization is present. Consequently, in relation to the articulatory apparatus involved in production, /r/ is more anterior than /l/. The feature [grave] will

[5] c.f. Lisker, "Minimal cues", 257, 262, 266 ff.

characterize this difference; /r/ is peripheral or [+ grave] in relation to /l/ which is central or [− grave].[6]

The revised description of liquids and semi-consonants is presented below:

	w	*y*	*r*	*l*
compact	−	+	−	−
grave	+	−	+	−

This analysis brings into sharp focus the relationships existing between the sound class semi-consonant (*w*,*y*) and liquids (*r*,*l*). The distinctive feature analysis implies that between these groups, the closest relationship exists between /w/ and /r/, and a looser bond exists between /y/ and /l/, /w/ and /l/, and /y/ and /r/. The data substantiates this description.

As indicated earlier, other frequent phoneme substitution errors occurring within the sonorant class were /n/ ↔ /l/ and /w/ ↔ /m/. The revised feature framework reflects this phenomenon. Thus,

	w	*y*	*r*	*l*	*m*	*n*	*ŋ*
compact	−	+	−	−	−	−	+
grave	+	−	+	−	+	−	+

As the chart indicates, both /n-l/ and /w-m/ are related by $\begin{bmatrix}\alpha \text{ compact} \\ \beta \text{ grave}\end{bmatrix}$ configurations, e.g. /n/ and /l/ are $\begin{bmatrix}- \text{ compact} \\ - \text{ grave}\end{bmatrix}$ and /w/ and /m/ are $\begin{bmatrix}- \text{ compact} \\ + \text{ grave}\end{bmatrix}$.

[6] It must be emphasized that the analysis of *r*—*l* presented above is restricted to English phonology. In other languages, the distinction between *r*—*l* by the feature [continuant] seems to be motivated on the basis of acoustic and articulatory criteria (c.f. Jakobson et al. (1962) 21). Consequently, although this analysis accounts for the aphasic data in English phonology it can not be used to describe the relationship between these two phonemes in other languages. Nevertheless, in all languages, the extremely close relationship between *r*—*l* is reflected universally by the late development of the distinction between these two phonemes in child language and their high frequency of confusions in aphasic speech. Thus, there seems to be a common feature underlying the representation of /r/ and /l/ in all languages which has not yet been fully captured in phonological theory. Therefore, the analysis proposed should be considered conjectural.

Consequently, the revised description can characterize simply and insightfully the close relationship felt between certain phoneme pairs within the class sonorant. Moreover, it not only accounts for the aphasic data but it also reflects sound relationships commonly found in child language acquisition and historical linguistics.

For a complete description of the class [sonorant], the features needed to distinguish its sub-classes, namely, semi-consonants, liquids, and nasals must also be specified. As the matrix now stands, there is no distinction made between these classes or the individual phonemes /w,r,m/ and /n,l/. According to the distinctive feature framework, these sub-classes can be differentiated by use of the features [consonantal], [vocalic], and [nasal]. Thus:

	w	*y*	*r*	*l*	*m*	*n*	*η*
sonorant	+	+	+	+	+	+	+
consonantal	–	–	+	+	+	+	+
vocalic	–	–	+	+	–	–	–
nasal	–	–	–	–	+	+	+
compact	–	+	–	–	–	–	+
grave	+	–	+	–	+	–	+

Note that within the sonorant class, the feature [nasal] distinguishes /m,n,η/ from semi-consonants /w,y/ and liquids /r,l/, and the features [consonantal] and [vocalic] distinguish /w,y/ from /r,l/.

In reviewing this matrix, an obvious difficulty can be noted – the relationship between semi-consonants and liquids, resonants, and nasals, so painstakingly characterized above is still described by a change involving the features [consonantal] and [vocalic]. Since these features are, so to speak, the most highly valued in the system, they should rarely be modified. As discussed earlier, the evidence from aphasia does not support this claim.

In order to account for the data, then, another solution is needed. One possible analysis is to mark the class of sonorants in some way so that a feature change involving [consonantal] or [vocalic] is evaluated as a minor rather than a highly marked sound change. However, not only is this restriction ad hoc but it also destroys the concept of the hierarchy. The hierarchical organization of the features reflects the stability or likelihood of a feature change and furthermore implies that a change at this level will critically modify the phoneme relationships within the phonological system.

Although not explicitly discussed, the solution to the problem is implicitly characterized in the phonological theories proposed by Jakobson et al. and Chomsky and Halle. The features [consonantal], [vocalic], and [sonorant] are classified by Jakobson as fundamental source features and by Chomsky and Halle as major class features.[7] This designation marks off the phonological system into three classes – consonant, vowel, and sonorant. It is in relation to these three major categories that the remaining features are presented. In this sense, then, the phonological system consists of three distinct sound classes, each of which consists of phonemes hierarchically organized according to the same phonological principles.

Indeed, there is an intuitive difference felt in the relationship between the classes of consonant, vowel, and sonorant, and the relationship of the phonemes belonging to these three classes. As the theory now stands, however, this difference is not explicitly expressed. Instead, features which define the three major classes are placed high on the hierarchy but are ostensibly equal in status to the remaining features in the system. Moreover, a sound change within a major class could be evaluated as equal in complexity to a change involving class membership. For example, the sound changes $\begin{bmatrix} w \\ p \end{bmatrix} \leftrightarrow \begin{bmatrix} r \\ u \end{bmatrix}$ both involve a change in the feature [consonantal] and [vocalic].

$$\begin{array}{ccccccc} w & \leftrightarrow & r & & p & \leftrightarrow & u \\ \begin{bmatrix} -\text{ cons.} \\ -\text{ voc.} \\ -\text{ comp.} \\ +\text{ grave} \end{bmatrix} & & \begin{bmatrix} +\text{ cons.} \\ +\text{ voc.} \\ -\text{ comp.} \\ +\text{ grave} \end{bmatrix} & & \begin{bmatrix} +\text{ cons.} \\ -\text{ voc.} \\ -\text{ comp.} \\ +\text{ grave} \end{bmatrix} & & \begin{bmatrix} -\text{ cons.} \\ +\text{ voc.} \\ -\text{ comp.} \\ +\text{ grave} \end{bmatrix} \end{array}$$

[7] c.f. Jakobson et al., *Preliminaries*, 18; Chomsky and Halle, *Sound Patterns*, 301 ff. Jakobson's classification of fundamental source features includes [consonantal] and [vocalic]. As mentioned earlier, he does not use the feature [sonorant] in his description.

Since this description in no way differentiates the reasonableness or likelihood of these two sound changes, it is considered inadequate.

In order to be able to characterize this important distinction, it is proposed that every sound within the system be marked for membership in at least one of the three classes – consonant, vowel, sonorant.[8] This classificatory feature would not be a part of the hierarchical arrangement of features but rather would stand in a dominance relation to them. Organized in this way, the theory would evaluate a change in a hierarchical feature and a class feature on two distinct levels – i.e. besides making a class feature change more highly marked than a hierarchical feature change and implying that such changes rarely occur, this dichotomy would express explicitly the difference between class changes as /d/ - /l/ and regular feature changes as /p/ - /t/.

This notion can be described within the present distinctive feature framework. The features [consonant] and [sonorant] define the three major classes; i.e.

[+ consonantal]	defines the consonants
[− consonantal]	defines the vowels
[+ sonorant]	defines the sonorants

Below this level, the distinctive differences are characterized hierarchically as before. Thus,

	p	*t*	*k*	*b*	*d*	*g*	*f*	*θ*	*s*	*š*	*v*	*δ*	*z*	*ž*	*č*	*ǰ*	*m*	*n*	*ŋ*	*w*	*y*	*r*	*l*	*h*	*V*
consonantal	+	+	+	+	+	+	+	+	+	+	+	+	+	+	+	+	+	+	+						−
sonorant																	+	+	+	+	+	+	+	+	
tense	+	+	+	−	−	−	+	+	+	+	−	−	−	−	+	−									
strident			−			−		−	+			−	+		+	+									
nasal	−	−	−	−	−	−	−	−	−	−	−	−	−	−	−	−	+	+	+	−	−	−	−	−	
grave	+	−		+	−		+	−	−		+	−	−				+	−		+	−	+	−	+	
compact	−	−	+	−	−	+	−	−	−	+	−	−	−	+	+	+	−	−	+	−	+	−	−	+	
contin.	−	−	−	−	−	−	+	+	+	+	+	+	+	+	−	−									
vocalic																				−	−	+	+	−	

[8] The nasal phonemes must be marked for membership in two major classes – consonant and sonorant. This will be discussed further in Chapter 8.

Note that the feature [vocalic] is used to define the distinctive difference between semi-consonants and liquids and elsewhere it is unspecified. Moreover, nasals are doubly marked as consonants and sonorants (this will be discussed in more detail in Chapter 8).

The level defined by major class features is further differentiated from the level below by the absence of binarily marked features to specify all class differences. Thus, consonants are defined as $\begin{bmatrix} + \text{C} \\ + \text{closed tract} \end{bmatrix}$ and vowels as $\begin{bmatrix} - \text{C} \\ - \text{closed tract} \end{bmatrix}$. Sonorants, on the other hand, define a class which is clearly subsidiary to both consonants and vowels, i.e. this class of phonemes contains features similar articulatorily, acoustically, and structurally to both [$\pm$ C]. This description implies that a more fundamental relationship exists between consonants and vowels, and sonorants, as a major class, are in some way different from but related to these two classes (for a complete discussion see Chapter 8).[9]

On the basis of this modified analysis, it is now possible to consider the remaining sound changes discussed earlier:

$$\begin{Bmatrix} t \\ d \end{Bmatrix} \leftrightarrow l \qquad \begin{Bmatrix} v \\ b \end{Bmatrix} \leftrightarrow w \qquad \begin{Bmatrix} k \\ g \end{Bmatrix} \leftrightarrow h$$

All these sound changes can be characterized by a class feature modification [+ consonant] $\leftrightarrow$ [+ sonorant]. Except for this difference, the features common to each sound share the same values. Hence:

[9] Although the introduction of the major class feature in the distinctive feature framework is well motivated, the adequacy and feasibility of the formal representation presented above may be questioned with regard to conditions of adequacy established by current phonological theory. However, the following analysis was made in an attempt to organize the data in some insightful way and to characterize the alleged psychological organization of the phonological system implied by the verbal behavior of aphasics, and not to devise an elaborate algebraic system based on excessively formal restrictions. Thus, however it may be represented formally, the notion major class feature should be considered an integral part of the phonological system of a language, and as a consequence, should be explicitly characterized in some way within a theoretical framework.

(1) $$l \quad \leftrightarrow \quad \begin{Bmatrix} d \\ t \end{Bmatrix}^{10}$$

$$\begin{bmatrix} + \text{ SONORANT} \\ - \text{ nasal} \\ - \text{ grave} \\ - \text{ compact} \\ \\ + \text{ vocalic} \end{bmatrix} \qquad \begin{bmatrix} + \text{ CONSONANT} \\ - \text{ nasal} \\ - \text{ grave} \\ - \text{ compact} \\ - \text{ continuant} \\ \\ \end{bmatrix}$$

(2) $$w \quad \leftrightarrow \quad \begin{Bmatrix} b \\ v \end{Bmatrix}$$

$$\begin{bmatrix} + \text{ SONORANT} \\ \\ - \text{ nasal} \\ + \text{ grave} \\ - \text{ compact} \\ - \text{ vocalic} \end{bmatrix} \qquad \begin{bmatrix} + \text{ CONSONANT} \\ - \text{ tense} \\ - \text{ nasal} \\ + \text{ grave} \\ - \text{ compact} \\ \\ \end{bmatrix}$$

(3) $$h \quad \leftrightarrow \quad \begin{Bmatrix} k \\ g \end{Bmatrix}$$

$$\begin{bmatrix} + \text{ SONORANT} \\ \\ - \text{ nasal} \\ + \text{ grave} \\ + \text{ compact} \\ \\ - \text{ vocalic} \end{bmatrix} \qquad \begin{bmatrix} + \text{ CONSONANT} \\ - \text{ strident} \\ - \text{ nasal} \\ \\ + \text{ compact} \\ - \text{ continuant} \\ \\ \end{bmatrix}$$

[10] It has been pointed out by S. Kuno (personal communication) that although the change from [+ consonant] → [+ sonorant] can account for the phonemic substitution of $\begin{Bmatrix} d \\ t \end{Bmatrix}$ → *l*, the reverse change, [+ sonorant] → [+ consonant] would fulfill the matrix specifications for /s, z, θ, ð/ as well as /t, d/; i.e. because /l/ is unspecified for continuancy, all $\begin{bmatrix} - \text{ nasal} \\ - \text{ grave} \\ - \text{ compact} \end{bmatrix}$ consonants would meet the distinctive feature description, and consequently, could theoretically be substituted for /l/. These consonants include /t, d, s, z, θ, ð/. However, the greater frequency of errors of l ↔ $\begin{Bmatrix} t \\ d \end{Bmatrix}$ in comparison to the rarety of errors between

Basic to the distinctive feature framework described above is the principle that all phonological units can be reduced to complexes of hierarchically ordered binary features. In 1954, Y. R. Chao questioned whether a dichotomous scale was, in fact, a principle inherent to the linguistic system.[11] Instead, he suggested that the notion of binary oppositions was merely a principle which could easily be imposed upon the structural system being analyzed. In reply to his critique, Jakobson discussed evidence from acquisition of language, and acoustic and articulatory experiments which seemed to support his original claim – namely, that the dichotomous scale is inherent to, not superimposed on, the phonological system of a language.[12] Evidence from aphasia would also seem to support this view.

In collecting the data for this study, it was observed that patients who could monitor their speech output would often make successive attempts at reaching the target word. For example,

	Attempts	Target
(1)	kədz → kən → kəmz	'comes'
(2)	tləd → pləd	'flood'
(3)	kiŋz → tiŋz	'things'
(4)	nEbələnd → nEdṛlənd	'Netherland'
(5)	θə → frIsən → prInstən	'Princeton'

In these examples, note that although the relationship between the error made in the first attempt and the target phoneme is defined

$l \leftrightarrow \begin{Bmatrix} s \\ z \\ \theta \\ \eth \end{Bmatrix}$ can be accounted for by the notion markedness. It seems reasonable to assume that if a substitution error occurs in which a major class feature is changed, that the substitution will involve the most unmarked phoneme within the given class. With regard to the class of consonants, stops are the most unmarked phonemes. Thus, it would be expected that the substitution of a $\begin{bmatrix} -\text{nasal} \\ -\text{grave} \\ -\text{compact} \end{bmatrix}$ consonant for a $\begin{bmatrix} -\text{nasal} \\ -\text{grave} \\ -\text{compact} \end{bmatrix}$ sonorant will occur with the unmarked consonants $\begin{Bmatrix} t \\ d \end{Bmatrix}$.

[11] Review of Jakobson, Halle, Fant, *Preliminaries to speech analysis*, *Romance Philology*, 8, 40–46 (1954) 44.

[12] *Fundamentals*, 47 ff.

by differences of more than one distinctive feature, the relationship between the phonemic errors made in each successive attempt is characterized by a single feature difference. Thus,

(1) *d* : *m* $\begin{bmatrix}\text{nasal}\\ \text{grave}\end{bmatrix}$ but *d* → *n* [nasal] → *m* [grave]

(2) *t* : *f* $\begin{bmatrix}\text{contin.}\\ \text{grave}\end{bmatrix}$ but *t* → *p* [grave] → *f* [contin.]

(3) *k* : θ $\begin{bmatrix}\text{contin.}\\ \text{compact}\end{bmatrix}$ but *k* → *t* [compact] → θ [contin.]

(4) *b* : δ $\begin{bmatrix}\text{grave}\\ \text{contin.}\end{bmatrix}$ but *b* → *d* [grave] → δ [contin.]

(5) θ : *p* $\begin{bmatrix}\text{contin.}\\ \text{grave}\end{bmatrix}$ but θ → *f* [grave] → *p* [contin.]

It is obvious from these examples that in the attempt to reach the target word, the patient is not arbitrarily substituting one phoneme for another. Instead, there seems to be a definite strategy underlying his verbal behavior. This strategy can best be characterized by the notion feature alteration, e.g. with each successive attempt, the phoneme substitution error is systematically modified by the alteration of a single feature value.

The feature alterations discussed above would seem to indicate that the strategy applied always results in a closer approximation to the target phoneme. This assumption, however, is stated too strongly. Numerous examples are found where the successive feature alterations bring the final verbal output away from the target phoneme. Compare:

Attempts			Target
(1) əta. . . → əsa . . .			'o'clock'
t : *k* [compact]	but *s* : *k*	$\begin{bmatrix}\text{contin.}\\ \text{compact}\end{bmatrix}$	
(2) pɔ → kɔ			'fall'
p : *k* [compact]	but *k* : *f*	$\begin{bmatrix}\text{contin.}\\ \text{compact}\end{bmatrix}$	
(3) dona → doda			'doña'
n : *ñ* [grave]	but *d* : *ñ*	$\begin{bmatrix}\text{nasal}\\ \text{grave}\end{bmatrix}$	

(4) ti ti → di ti 'P. T.'

t : *p* [grave] but *d* : *p* $\begin{bmatrix}\text{grave}\\ \text{tense}\end{bmatrix}$

(5) dəst → nəst 'just'

d : *ǰ* [compact] but *n* : *ǰ* $\begin{bmatrix}\text{nasal}\\ \text{compact}\end{bmatrix}$

Despite the fact that this strategy is, so to speak, incorrectly developed, the notion feature alteration described earlier can still be maintained; namely, with each successive attempt, only one feature specification is altered at a time.

It is this notion of feature alteration which strongly suggests that the dichotomous scale is more than a description imposed on language structure. Rather, it would seem that this phenomenon not only exhibits the intrinsic nature of the binary features to the phonological system of the language but also suggests that binarily coded features may be a basic notion in a model for speech production.

8

SOME ASPECTS OF MARKEDNESS

The theory of markedness has been of increasing importance in current phonological theory. According to the theoretical framework established, the direction of one distinctive feature substitution errors made by aphasics should be from marked to unmarked. The analysis of the aphasic data supported this claim – there was a greater tendency for unmarked consonants to be substituted for marked consonants rather than the reverse.

If it is assumed that the directionality of substitution errors reveals the underlying markedness relationships of the phonological system, then it may be possible to look to the aphasic data for evidence concerning the markedness relationships between phonological pairs which have not been clearly established in phonological theory. Such a case is found between the phoneme pairs $\begin{bmatrix} \text{p}-\text{t} \\ \text{b}-\text{d} \end{bmatrix}$.

As Chomsky and Halle have stated ,"In view of the fact that the unmarked nasal must be /n/ and the unmarked continuant /s/, the unmarked plosive – if there were to be one – would have to be /t/. This conclusion, however, seems unacceptable to us; in particular, the choice of the dental over the labial plosive appears incorrect."[1]. The preference for the labial consonant seems to stem primarily from evidence of child language acquisition. Here, labials seem to be acquired before dentals. Thus, in his monograph *Child Language, Aphasia, and Phonological Universals*, Jakobson says " ... The following laws are thus explained all at once: the priority of the labial consonant and the a-vowel; the priority of the basic line in

[1] *Sound Patterns*, 413.

the consonantal system . . . , i.e. the priority of the split of oral and nasal consonants into labial and dental . . ."[2]

An analysis of the substitution errors made between $\begin{bmatrix} p-t \\ b-d \end{bmatrix}$ in aphasic speech may give some insight into the solution of this problem. The mean percent of errors made in the direction $\begin{bmatrix} p \\ b \end{bmatrix} \rightarrow \begin{bmatrix} t \\ d \end{bmatrix}$ and $\begin{bmatrix} t \\ d \end{bmatrix} \rightarrow \begin{bmatrix} p \\ b \end{bmatrix}$ is seen below. These percentages are based on raw scores of 36 and 17 errors for Broca's, and Conduction aphasics respectively. Since the Wernicke distribution is based on only one example, no conclusions can be drawn from this sample.

	Broca's	Conduction
$\begin{bmatrix} p \\ b \end{bmatrix} \rightarrow \begin{bmatrix} t \\ d \end{bmatrix}$	46 %	28 %
$\begin{bmatrix} t \\ d \end{bmatrix} \rightarrow \begin{bmatrix} p \\ b \end{bmatrix}$	54 %	72 %

The distributions demonstrated by the Broca's and Conduction aphasics suggest a tendency for errors to go from dental → labial consonants. If, on the basis of the previous analysis, it is assumed that the direction of consonant errors goes from marked → unmarked, then the greater number of dental → labial errors suggests that the labial plosives are the unmarked and dental plosives are the marked consonants of the phonological system.

These results are interesting in light of the relationship between the nasals homorganic to these stops, i.e. m-n. The criteria used for determining markedness relations hold that within the class of nasals, /n/ is the unmarked phoneme.[3] In the distinctive feature analysis of nasals, /m/ is distinguished from /n/ by the feature [grave]. Thus, /m/, the marked phoneme, is [+ grave] and /n/, the unmarked phoneme, is [− grave]. Within the class of stops, the feature [grave] is also used to distinguish /p/ from /t/, /p/ is

[2] 77ff.

[3] For discussion of this question see: Chomsky and Halle, *Sound Patterns*, 413; C. Ferguson, "Assumptions about nasals: a sample study in phonological universals", in *Universals of Language*, ed. J. Greenberg (Cambridge, 1963) 56; R. Jakobson, "Mufaxxama, the 'emphatic' phonemes in Arabic", in *Selected Writings*, I, (The Hague, 1962) 514ff.; Trubetzkoy, *Grundzüge*, 193.

[+ grave] and /t/ is [− grave]. However, as shown above, /p/, [+ grave], is the unmarked phoneme, and /t/, [− grave], is the marked phoneme. Thus, there is a dissociation between the + or − value of the feature and the markedness value assigned to it, e.g. [+grave] is the unmarked value of the feature within the class of stops distinguishing /p/ from /t/, and it is the marked value within the class of nasals distinguishing /m/ from /n/.

This dissociation demonstrates that markedness relations are not always reflected by the particular binary value assigned to a feature, i.e. + does not always mean marked and − unmarked. Instead, there is a complex bond between the distinctive feature specification and markedness relations. The feature specifications define phonemic relationships within the system. However, $\{^{+}_{-}\}$ values of the features do not necessarily reflect the hierarchical relationship between the phonemes defined by them. Rather, it is the notion markedness which characterizes this hierarchical organization. Thus, an insightful description of the phonological system of a language cannot be made without reference to both of these notions.

Within the major class features introduced in Chapter 7, ther is also a hierarchical organization which can be described in terms of markedness. Thus, a complete phonological description of the notion major class must necessarily include the feature specifications used as well as the markedness relationships between class members.

The features [consonant] and [sonorant] define the three major classes – consonant, vowel, and sonorant. Evidence from aphasic speech and linguistics proper indicates that the features [consonant] and [sonorant] are not equally marked. Instead, [consonant] seems to be basic to the phonological system while the feature [sonorant] stands in a secondary or subordinate relation to it.

Firstly, consonants and vowels are the first major class distinctions acquired by the child. The phonemes comprising the sonorant class are relatively late acquisitions in the child's phonemic inventory. On this basis alone, the phonological system of the language seems to be divided primarily into consonants ([+ consonantal]) and vowels ([– consonantal]), and only secondarily into sonorants.

Moreover, this organization is reflected in all areas of linguistics including psychological studies of normal and pathological speech, historical linguistics, and dialectology. It is a common fact that consonants and vowels tend to maintain their distinctiveness in relation to each other. This is not the case with sonorants. As discussed in Chapter 7, examples abound in the literature where sonorants are confused with or substituted for consonants.

It is for these reasons that the major class features are felt to be hierarchically organized. The unmarked feature [consonant] defines the two major classes and consequently, the basic dichotomy of the phonological system – consonants and vowels. The marked major class feature [sonorant] defines a class of phonemes distinct from, but subordinate to, the feature [consonant].

Although [sonorant] may be subordinate to the feature [consonant], it is not clear whether this relationship is equally reflected within the classes defined by [consonant], i.e. whether the class [sonorant] is distinct from but subordinate to consonants ([+ consonant]), on the one hand, and vowels ([– consonant]), on the other.

The relationship between consonants and sonorants is much more obvious than that between sonorants and vowels. In the first place, it is generally recognized in linguistics that consonants and sonorants are commonly substituted for each other (see Chapter 7). Moreover, a clear link between these two classes is established by the description of the class of nasal phonemes. On the basis of acoustic and articulatory criteria, as well as structural considerations, nasals are doubly marked for membership in the class of sonorants and class of consonants. As sonorants, nasals are intimately linked with liquids and semi-consonants; as consonants, they are intimately linked to tense and lax stops. An analysis of the errors involving this dual class clearly demonstrates the nature of the relationship between consonants and sonorants.

Only those nasal phoneme substitution errors which clearly reflected membership in either the consonant or sonorant class were used in this analysis. The analysis of errors made is summarized below:

MAJOR CLASS	ERROR TYPES	% FOR APHASIC SAMPLE
[+ consonant]	nasal – {tense / lax} stops	62.8 %
[+ sonorant]	nasal – {liquids / semi-*C*}	37.2 %

These percentages, based on a total of 129 errors, indicate that more errors occurred when nasals were marked as [+ consonant], i.e. between nasals and stops, and fewer errors occurred when nasals were marked [+ sonorant], i.e. between nasals and liquids or semi-consonants. In Chapter 4, it was shown that the frequency of errors made between phonemes was positively correlated with the closeness of the bond existing between them. Thus, the fact that more nasal substitution errors occurred with consonants than sonorants suggests that nasals are more intrinsically related to the major class consonant than to the major class sonorant. This relationship is characterized by the hypothesized organization of major class features – consonants are unmarked and sonorants are marked.

The relationship between vowels and sonorants is not as obvious. Perhaps the most obvious similarity between these two classes is based on distributional features. In English, sonorants become syllabic peaks in interconsonantal position or following a consonant in final position; for example, [bṛd] 'bird', [bəʔṇ] 'button', [baɾḷ] 'bottle'. Thus, in these environments, sonorants and vowels are in contrasting environments – c.p. [bṛd]–[bId] 'bird'–'bid', [baɾḷ]–[baɾi] 'bottle'–'body'. In this sense, then, sonorants have a certain relation to vowels that consonants do not have. Moreover, although sonorants were never confused with pure vowels in the aphasic data, several examples were found where syllabic sonorants became *V* + sonorant, e.g. [hṛd] 'heard' → [hɔrd], [bṛn] 'burn' → [birn], and vice versa, e.g. [varsIti] 'varsity' → [fṛ . . .] → [farsIti], [pær] 'pear' → [pṛ]. Examples of this type suggest that the vocalic nature of these syllables is inherent to this class of phonemes.

In addition, an investigation of the acoustic and articulatory factors involved in the production of sonorants in English shows the dual nature of this class of phonemes, i.e. sonorants combine distinctive traits of both consonants and vowels.

In acoustic analysis, it can be seen that the formant structure of sonorants is vocalic in nature. However, variations in direction and extent of formant 2 and 3 seem to be cues for the perception of place of production for stops, nasals, liquids, and semi-consonants while comparable variations of formant 1 are cues for manner, i.e. stops vs. nasals vs. liquids vs. semi-consonants.[4] These transitions are consonantal qualities and are not found in the acoustic representation of vowels.

The articulation of sonorants is neither completely vocalic in nature – characterized by free passage of air in the oral cavity, nor is it completely consonantal – characterized by occlusion or friction in the oral cavity. The production of liquids (*r,l*) is characterized by free passage of air around either a medial or lateral obstruction. Nasals (*m,n,ŋ*) are characterized by closure in the oral cavity with free flow of air through the nasal cavity. Finally, glides (*w,y*) are produced by ballistic movements in the oral cavity, thus resulting in neither a free flow of air nor obstruction of air in the oral cavity.

On the basis of the evidence presented above drawn from all areas of linguistics – child language, aphasia, historical linguistics, and acoustic and articulatory phonetics, it is concluded that the class sonorant is distinct from but subordinate to both consonants [+ consonantal] and vowels [– consonantal], and consequently, the major class feature [sonorant] is marked and the feature [consonantal] is unmarked.

[4] Liberman, "Speech perception", 144.

9

DISTINCTIVE AND REDUNDANT FEATURES

The linguistic investigation of aphasic speech has to this point dealt exclusively with the distinctive features of the phonological system – i.e. those features which are used to distinguish one phoneme from another within the system. However, evidence from the aphasic data has suggested that the distinctive values alone may not be able to account for all of the phonological errors made in aphasic speech.

An analysis of the relationship between the stop consonants and their homorganic nasals revealed that consistently more phoneme substitution errors occurred between lax stops and their homorganic nasals than tense stops and nasals; for example, the substitution $m \leftrightarrow b$ occurred more frequently than $m \leftrightarrow p$. Thus,

	Broca	Conduction	Wernicke
Nasal $\sim C_{lax}$	72.3 %	76.7 %	66.7 %
Nasal $\sim C_{tense}$	27.7 %	23.3 %	33.3 %

The mean percents obtained are based on raw scores of 67, 11, and 3 for Broca's, Conduction, and Wernicke's aphasics respectively. Although the figures for Wernicke's aphasics are too small to make any conclusions, the general similarities among the aphasic groups are striking.

Intuitively, this pattern does not seem at all surprising. Nasals are lax consonants and consequently, should be more closely related to lax stops than tense stops. However, on the phonemic level, this distinction is not expressed. Because tenseness is a redundant feature for nasals, it is unspecified on the phonemic level;

thus, lax and tense stops are distinguished from nasals only by the feature [nasal]. The greater similarity between nasals and lax consonants is not specified until the redundant features are expressed. Then, a comparison of the fully specified matrices indicates that lax consonants and nasals are differentiated by only one feature [nasal], and tense consonants and nasals are differentiated by two features – [tense] and [nasal].

Similar patterns were found between $\begin{Bmatrix}\text{tense}\\\text{lax}\end{Bmatrix}$ consonants and those phonemes unspecified for voicing on the phonemic level. Compare the following raw scores:

	Broca	Conduction	Wernicke
t-l	2	2	0
d-l	10	1	2
p-w	0	0	0
b-w	24	2	1
f-w	1	3	0
v-w	18	1	0
k-h	5	8	1
g-h	2	0	0

The fact that, in general, more errors occur between those phonemes equally marked for tenseness (c.p. $\begin{Bmatrix}t\\d\end{Bmatrix} - l$ and $\begin{Bmatrix}k\\g\end{Bmatrix} - h$) suggests that these substitution errors may be based on redundant features as well as distinctive features. If errors occurred only at the level where distinctive differences are expressed, then it would be expected that substitution errors would occur as frequently between lax consonants and their respective sonorants as between tense consonants and sonorants. If, on the other hand, substitution errors occurred based on redundant features as well as distinctive features, then the greater frequency of errors between lax consonants and sonorants would be accounted for simply by a single feature change as compared to a two feature change for an error between tense consonants and sonorants.

The possibility that phonological errors can occur based on

redundant features as well as distinctive features has important implications for linguistic theory. Before considering them, however, it is necessary to determine whether there are other examples of errors in the aphasic data which clearly reflect the need for different levels of analysis.

In English, vowels are nasalized when they precede nasal consonants in closed syllables. Because the nasalization of vowels is always predictable from the environment, nasalized vowels are nonphonemic. Thus, low level redundancy rules describe the assimilation of the nasality feature of the consonant to the preceding vowel. For example, the vowel /æ/ in 'hand' is not nasalized on the phonemic level. However, it is interpreted phonetically as a nasalized vowel – /hænd/ 'hand', [hæ̃nd]. This suggests a given order for the derivation of the lexical item:

(1) phonemic representation / V N/
+ nasal

(A) nasal assimilation V N
+ nasal + nasal

(2) phonetic representation [Ṽ N]

In the aphasic data, many examples of the loss of nasal consonants were found. An analysis of the vowels preceding these consonants provides evidence for determining where in the derivation of the lexical item the nasal consonant was lost. If, on the one hand, the vowel preceding the nasal consonant were not nasalized, then the consonant loss occurred before nasal assimilation. The vowel would then be interpreted phonetically as an oral vowel. If, on the other hand, the vowel were nasalized, then the nasal consonant could only have been lost after the nasality feature was assimilated to the preceding vowel.

The difference between these two processes can be seen by the following diagram:

(a) simplification before assimilation	(b) simplification after assimilation
(1) / V N /	(1) / V N /
+ nasal	+ nasal
↓ ø	
(A) Nasal assimilation cannot apply	(A) V N
	+ nasal + nasal (↑ ___ ↓ ø)
(2) [V]	(2) [Ṽ]

A review of the data indicates that consonant simplifications occurred both before and after nasal assimilation. Compare:

(a)		(b)	
wɔlθə	'Waltham'	mə̃di	'Monday'
rɔ → lɔ	'lawn'	fæ̃wi	'family'
frIsə̃n	'Princeton'	bEbĨ	'heaven'
peit	'paint'	præ̃	'plant'
sig	'sing'	kə̃viuz	'confuse'

In (a), the vowels preceding the lost nasal consonants were not nasalized, indicating that the simplification of the consonant occurred before nasal assimilation. In (b), the nasalized vowels indicate that the loss of the consonant occurred after nasal assimilation. Examples of both types of errors were found in the speech production of the same patient, indicating that one type of error was not restricted to some patients and another type to others.

Similar findings were found in the simplification of the clusters $/\# s \left\{\begin{matrix}p\\t\\k\end{matrix}\right\}/$. In English, the allophones of /p,t,k/ are voiceless and unaspirated when they follow initial/s/, i.e. $/\# s \left\{\begin{matrix}p\\t\\k\end{matrix}\right\}/$, $[\# s \left\{\begin{matrix}p^-\\t^-\\k^-\end{matrix}\right\}]$. Thus, the phonetic interpretation of /p,t,k/ is directly dependent on the occurrence of the preceding /s/. With the loss of this initial

/s/ in aphasic speech, two types of examples were found. In the first, /p,t,k/ were voiceless and unaspirated; for example, 'speech' → [p⁻ič], 'special' → [p⁻Ešəl]. In the second, /p,t,k/ were voiceless and aspirated; for example, 'scholarship' → [k^hal . . .], 'scotch' → [k^hač]. These examples suggest that the loss of /s/ occurs at different points in the derivation of the lexical item. In the first, the cluster was simplified after /p,t,k/ were interpreted phonetically as part of the cluster /# s $\left\{\begin{matrix}p\\t\\k\end{matrix}\right\}$ /. Thus:

(1) phonemic representation /# s $\left\{\begin{matrix}p\\t\\k\end{matrix}\right\}$ /

(2) phonetic representation [# s $\left\{\begin{matrix}p^-\\t^-\\k^-\end{matrix}\right\}$] → [# $\left\{\begin{matrix}p^-\\t^-\\k^-\end{matrix}\right\}$]

In the second, the cluster was simplified before the phonetic interpretation of the lexical item. Thus, /p,t,k/ were interpreted phonetically as initial stops:[1]

[1] Although these errors suggest that phonological errors occur on several levels of analysis, it must be emphasized that this interpretation is based on a particular theoretical bias, namely that the allophones [p⁻, t⁻, k⁻] belong to the phonemes /p, t, k/ respectively. It is not altogether certain that [p⁻, t⁻, k⁻] should be assigned to /p, t, k/ instead of /b, d, g/. The assignment of [p⁻, t⁻, k⁻] to /p, t, k/ seems to be based primarily on English orthography rather than on any compelling linguistic evidence. In fact, since the stop consonants become lax, i.e. unaspirated, in the position of neutralization, it could be argued that these consonants should be assigned to the lax stop consonants, i.e. /b, d, g/. Moreover, regardless of the phoneme these allophones are assigned to in descriptive analysis, it is unclear whether the sounds are considered psychologically as tense or lax stops, or, in fact, if their membership is clearly defined. Further evidence from the aphasic data suggests that in positions of neutralization, there may not be consistent assignment of an allophone to a specific phoneme. This evidence is based on the phoneme substitution errors for /t/ and /d/ in intervocalic position. In this environment, /t/ and d/ become neutralized, i.e. $\left\{\begin{matrix}t\\d\end{matrix}\right\}$ → ɾ. Compare:

/lEtəs/ 'lettuce' [lEɾəs]
/mIdəl/ 'middle' [mIɾl̩]

In the aphasic data, there was a relatively large number of two distinctive feature substitution errors made for /t/ in intervocalic position; for example, /lEtr/'letter' → [lEδr̩], /gətrz/ 'gutters' → [gəδr̩z], /bətrflai/ butterfly' → [bəvə . . .]. Note, however, that in these examples, there is only a one distinctive feature difference

(1) phonemic representation $/\#\, s \left\{\begin{matrix}p\\t\\k\end{matrix}\right\} / \rightarrow /\# \left\{\begin{matrix}p\\t\\k\end{matrix}\right\} /$

(2) phonetic representation $[\# \left\{\begin{matrix}p^h\\t^h\\k^h\end{matrix}\right\}]$

One further class of errors suggests the importance of redundant as well as distinctive features in the phonological analysis of aphasic speech. This error type involves the range of substitution errors occurring with the phonemes $\left\{\begin{matrix}\check{c}\\\check{j}\end{matrix}\right\}$. Although these sounds are phonetically equivalent to the clusters $\left[\begin{matrix}t + \check{s}\\d + \check{z}\end{matrix}\right]$, their structural distribution suggests that they be analyzed as unit phonemes. An analysis of the distribution of errors made with these phonemes sheds some light on whether $\left\{\begin{matrix}\check{c}\\\check{j}\end{matrix}\right\}$ is considered psychologically for the speaker as a unit phoneme or cluster. From these results, important conclusions can be drawn concerning the features involved in substitution errors with these phonemes.

Two types of substitution errors occur with the phonemes $\left\{\begin{matrix}\check{c}\\\check{j}\end{matrix}\right\}$. In the first, $\left\{\begin{matrix}\check{c}\\\check{j}\end{matrix}\right\}$ and a single consonant are substituted for each other, e.g. $\check{c} \rightarrow C$, /čIldrən/ 'children' → /tIldrən/, /məč/ 'much' → /mək/; $C \rightarrow \check{c}$, /šEl/ 'shell' → /čEl/, /fiučr̩/ 'future' → /fiušr̩/. In the second, $\left\{\begin{matrix}\check{c}\\\check{j}\end{matrix}\right\}$ and a consonant cluster are substituted for each other, e.g. $\check{c} \rightarrow C_1C_2$, /tič/ 'teach' → /tits/, /məč/ 'much' →

---

between the substitution errors and /d/. These results suggest that the assignment of [ɾ] to /t/ in the above examples may not be clearly defined psychologically as the linguistic analysis would imply. As in the case of the clusters $/\#s \left\{\begin{matrix}p\\t\\k\end{matrix}\right\}/$, the assignment of [ɾ] to the particular phoneme /t/ or /d/ seems to be based primarily on English orthography. It is interesting to note that in all cases of substitutions for [ð] occurring at morpheme boundaries, all errors were one distinctive feature from the underlying phoneme representation; for example, [weikən] 'waiting' and [riðiŋ] 'reading'. Although the phonemes /t/ and /d/ were neutralized in these environments, the phonemic representation is clearly defined by the underlying morphemic representation – {weit} 'wait', {rid} 'read'. On the basis of this evidence, it is suggested that the analysis of /p, t, k/ presented above be considered speculative in nature.

/məts/; $C_1C_2 \rightarrow$ č, /šits/ 'sheets' $\rightarrow$ /šič/, /bits/ 'beets' $\rightarrow$ /bič/. It would seem that the errors involving $\begin{Bmatrix} \check{c} \\ \check{j} \end{Bmatrix}$ and a single consonant can be used as evidence for $\begin{Bmatrix} \check{c} \\ \check{j} \end{Bmatrix}$ being unit phonemes and those involving $\begin{Bmatrix} \check{c} \end{Bmatrix}$ and two consonants, evidence for $\begin{Bmatrix} \check{c} \\ \check{j} \end{Bmatrix}$ being clusters.

An analysis of the environmental distribution of each error type, however, reveals crucial differences. Errors involving $\begin{Bmatrix} \check{c} \\ \check{j} \end{Bmatrix} \rightarrow C$ are found in initial, medial, and final position; whereas, 17 out of 18 errors involving $\begin{Bmatrix} \check{c} \\ \check{j} \end{Bmatrix} \rightarrow C_1C_2$ occur only in final position. Moreover, out of these 17 errors, 15 of them included substitutions between $\begin{Bmatrix} \check{c} \\ \check{j} \end{Bmatrix}$ and $\begin{Bmatrix} ts \\ dz \end{Bmatrix}$. Thus, the distribution of errors are in contrasting environments only in word final position.

Because of the frequency of substitutions between $\begin{Bmatrix} \check{c} \\ \check{j} \end{Bmatrix}$ and $\begin{Bmatrix} ts \\ dz \end{Bmatrix}$, it is interesting to note the distribution of $\begin{Bmatrix} ts \\ dz \end{Bmatrix}$ in English. Although /ts/ occurs in initial, medial, and final position, its distribution initially and medially is restricted to learned words, e.g. tsar, matzo; names, Fitzimmon; or at morpheme boundaries, e.g. outside, artsy. The distribution of /dz/, on the other hand, seems limited to names, e.g. Godzilla, and plurals in word final position. e.g. cards. Consequently, the substitution of $\begin{Bmatrix} ts \\ dz \end{Bmatrix}$ for $\begin{Bmatrix} \check{c} \\ \check{j} \end{Bmatrix}$ in initial or medial position would result in either marginally acceptable or completely unacceptable English phonological sequences. It has been observed that very few of the total phonological errors made by aphasics break the allowable English sequence constraints (see Chapter 5).

The fact that errors involving $\begin{Bmatrix} \check{c} \\ \check{j} \end{Bmatrix}$ and two consonants have such a restricted environmental distribution, and as a result of this restriction, maintain the rules of English phonology strongly suggests that $\begin{Bmatrix} \check{c} \\ \check{j} \end{Bmatrix}$ are psychologically unit phonemes. Moreover, if $\begin{Bmatrix} \check{c} \\ \check{j} \end{Bmatrix}$ were considered phonemically as the clusters $\begin{bmatrix} t + \check{s} \\ d + \check{z} \end{bmatrix}$, then errors with $\begin{bmatrix} t + \check{s} \\ d + \check{z} \end{bmatrix}$ and $\begin{Bmatrix} t \\ d \end{Bmatrix}$ would have to be accounted for by phonemic loss, e.g. /tšIldrən/ 'children' → /tIldrən/, and errors between $\begin{bmatrix} t + \check{s} \\ d + \check{z} \end{bmatrix}$ and $\begin{Bmatrix} k \\ g \end{Bmatrix}$ could not be accounted for at all within the distinctive feature framework, e.g. /džṛməni/ 'Germany' → /gṛməni/, /gṛl/ 'girl' → /džṛl/, /mətš/ 'much' → /mək/. However, considered phonemically as unit phonemes, substitution errors between $\begin{Bmatrix} \check{c} \\ \check{j} \end{Bmatrix}$ and $\begin{Bmatrix} k \\ g \end{Bmatrix}$, $\begin{Bmatrix} t \\ d \end{Bmatrix}$, $\begin{Bmatrix} \check{s} \\ \check{z} \end{Bmatrix}$, can be accounted for simply by single feature changes of [strident], [compact], and [continuant], respectively.

With the unit phoneme as a premise, it is necessary to see if errors between $\begin{Bmatrix} \check{c} \\ \check{j} \end{Bmatrix}$ and two consonants can be accounted for. As indicated earlier, nearly all errors between $\begin{Bmatrix} \check{c} \\ \check{j} \end{Bmatrix}$ and consonant clusters involved $\begin{bmatrix} ts \\ dz \end{bmatrix}$. A comparison of the articulation of these sounds demonstrates the similarity between them – both *ts* and *č* are tense, strident, non-continuants. They differ only in point of articulation – the sequence *ts* is pronounced with the blade of the tongue more forward than the position of the tongue in the articulation of *č*. Thus, in the fully specified matrix for *č*, a change of compactness from [+ compact] to [– compact] will result in the bundle of features which are phonetically equivalent to the sequence *ts*. Compare:

	č	*ts*
consonant	+	+
tense	+	+
strident	+	+
nasal	–	–
grave	–	–
compact	+	–
contin.	–	–
vocalic	–	–

However, it was stated above that the substitution of *č* → *t* is also described by a single feature change of [+ compact] to [– compact]. Thus, according to these two analyses, compactness distinguishes *č* and *t*, on the one hand, and *č* and *ts*, on the other. This apparent discrepancy can be accounted for by considering the level on which the feature change occurred.

On the phonemic level, the distinctive feature matrices for *č* and *t* are:

	č	*t*
consonant	+	+
tense	+	+
strident	+	
compact	+	–
contin.	–	–

Note that /t/ is distinguished from /č/ by the feature [compact], and also, that /t/ is unspecified for stridency. The feature [strident] is redundant for the phoneme /t/. However, in the fully specified matrix, /t/ will be marked for stridency, e.g. [– strident]. Thus, on the phonemic level, /č/ is distinguished from /t/ by only one feature – [compact]. However, when all features are specified in the matrix, /č/ and /t/ are no longer distinguished by one feature. Compare:

	č	*t*
consonant	+	+
tense	+	+
strident	+	–
nasal	–	–
grave	–	–
compact	+	–
contin.	–	–
vocalic	–	–

Note that they are distinguished now by two features – stridency and compactness.

Thus, on the level of autonomous distinctions, a change in the feature [compact] will result in the substitution of *č-t*. However, when redundant features as well as the distinctive features are expressed, a change in the feature [compact] will result in the substitution of *č-ts*.

The analysis of *č-ts* substitutions as sub-phonemic feature changes, i.e. errors based on both distinctive and redundant features, is supported by considerations of the direction that *č-ts* errors take. In the aphasic data, twice as many substitution errors occurred between *č* and *ts* (10), i.e. $\check{c} \rightarrow ts$, than between *ts* and *č* (5), i.e. $ts \rightarrow \check{c}$. It will be remembered that nearly all of these errors occurred in word final position. In English, the occurrence of non-continuant stridents in word final position is nearly always realized phonetically as the sequence [stop + $\begin{Bmatrix} s \\ z \end{Bmatrix}$] – c.p. the English plurals $C + \begin{Bmatrix} s \\ z \end{Bmatrix}$ #. Consequently, it would be expected that substitution errors will be directed by the greater frequency of $\begin{Bmatrix} s \\ z \end{Bmatrix}$ in comparison to $\begin{Bmatrix} \check{s} \\ \check{z} \end{Bmatrix}$ in word final position.

Now that it has been established that substitution errors can occur based on redundant features as well as distinctive features, it is necessary to return to the original problem, namely, can the greater frequency of errors between lax consonants and sonorants be triggered by the fact that they share a redundant feature [– tense]. On the basis of the examples discussed above, it seems that phonological errors do occur on several levels. Consequently, the analysis of $\begin{Bmatrix} \text{nasals} \\ \text{liquids} \end{Bmatrix}$ and $\begin{Bmatrix} \text{tense} \\ \text{lax} \end{Bmatrix}$ consonants based on the specification of redundant features seems to be a motivated and reasonable interpretation of the data.

These results have important implications for current phonological theory. According to current generative phonological theory the intrinsic relationships among the phonemes of the language are expressed on the systematic phonemic level. Morpheme structure rules and phonological rules fill in all redundant features. The fully specified matrix is represented on the phonetic level. On this level, every feature is of equal value, i.e. the underlying relationships expressed on the systematic phonemic level are now no longer represented.

Evidence from aphasia suggests that this approach to phonology is not only counterintuitive, but it also ignores the fact that BOTH the phonemic and phonetic levels are bound together as part of a language system – a system whose parts are not strictly separated but rather complexly interrelated.

It would seem that the speaker defines his phonological system in terms of the implicit relationships defined on the phonemic level. These relationships remain constant regardless of whether the phonological matrix is fully specified or not. For example, it would seem that, for the speaker, *p-m* are intrinsically related in a way that *d-m* are not, regardless of the fact that in the fully specified matrix, i.e. on the phonetic level, both sound pairs are distinguished by the same number of distinctive features – *p-m* by $\begin{bmatrix}\text{voice}\\ \text{nasal}\end{bmatrix}$ and *d-m* by $\begin{bmatrix}\text{grave}\\ \text{nasal}\end{bmatrix}$.

This view stands to reason if one considers what these relationships mean in terms of the speaker of the language. On the phonemic level, the relationships among the phonemes of the language are defined. This results in a particular psychological bond – i.e. for each phoneme pair, a particular bond is established; the closer the phonological relationship, the closer the bond. Once this bond is established, it spans the entire language system. As a consequence, the nature and direction of phonological errors made are a direct function of the psychological bond established on the phonemic level, regardless of the particular level on which the errors occur.

10

SUMMARY

The phonological investigation of aphasic speech has not only served as a testing ground for theoretical linguistic assumptions but it has also contributed some additional insights into phonological theory.

The notion distinctive feature has provided a principled explanation for the frequency of the different types of substitution errors made by aphasics. Errors occurred most frequently between phonemes related by one distinctive feature and fewer errors occurred between phonemes separated by more than one distinctive feature.

Although a majority of errors were characterized by the distinctive feature framework, a small group of 'exceptions' consistently occurred. This group of errors was found to be systematically described by the addition of the feature sonorant to the distinctive feature framework and the division of the framework into major class features and hierarchical features.

Further analysis of the data revealed that phonological errors were based on redundant features as well as distinctive features. These results suggested that regardless of whether an error was based on distinctive or redundant features, the nature and direction of the phonological errors made were a direct function of the psychological bond – i.e. the nature of the phonological relationship – established on the level of autonomous distinctive features. Moreover, the strategies for speech production demonstrated by aphasic patients suggested that the binary values ascribed to features in phonological theory may be an intrinsic part of the phonological system of the speaker.

In addition to the notion distinctive feature, the notion markedness proved to be an essential aspect of phonological analysis. The notion markedness characterized the direction of substitution and simplification errors made by aphasics – i.e. marked phonological structures and syllable structures tended to become unmarked. Moreover, evidence from the aphasic data suggested that $\begin{Bmatrix} p \\ b \end{Bmatrix}$ are the unmarked consonants of the stop consonant series and that within the major class features, consonant is the unmarked feature and sonorant the marked feature. It is the notion markedness which is able to elucidate the complex network of phoneme class and phoneme class relationships comprising the phonological system of the language. Thus, markedness serves to complement the insights made by the concept distinctive feature concerning phonological organization. Neither alone can adequately describe all the linguistic facts brought to bear in this study. However, together they account for a substantial portion of the data simply and insightfully.

REFERENCES

Alajouanine, T., A. Ombredane and M. Durand
1939 *Le Syndrome de la Désintégration Phonétique dans l'Aphasie* (Paris, Masson).

Blumstein, S.
1968 "Phonological aspects of aphasic speech", in *Studies Presented to Professor R. Jakobson by his Students*, ed. C. Gribble (Cambridge, Slavica) 39–43.
1970 *Phonological Implications of Aphasic Speech*, unpublished doctoral dissertation, Harvard University.

Bouman, L. and A. Grünbaum
1925 "Experimentell-psychologische untersuchungen zur aphasie und paraphasie", *Zeitschrift für die gesamte Neurologie und Psychiatrie*, 96, 481–538.

Chao, Y. R.
1954 "Review of Jakobson, Halle, Fant, *Preliminaries to speech analysis*", *Romance Philology*, 8, 1, 40–46.

Chomsky, N. and M. Halle
1968 *The Sound Pattern of English* (New York, Harper & Row).

Cohen, D., J. Dubois, M. Gauthier, H. Hécaen, and R. Angelergues
1963 "Aspects du fonctionnement du code linguistique chez les aphasiques moteurs", *Neuropsychologia*, 1, 165–177.

Critchley, M.
1952 "Articulatory defects in aphasia", *Journal of Laryngology and Otology*, 66, 1–17.

Denes, P. B.
1963 "On the statistics of spoken English", *Journal of the Acoustical Society of America*, 35, 892–904.

Dubois, J., H. Hécaen, R, Angelergues, M. Chatelier and P. Marcie
1964 "Etude neurolinguistique de l'aphasie de conduction", *Neuropsychologia*, 2, 9–44.

Ferguson, C.
1963 "Assumptions about nasals : a sample study in phonological universals", in *Universals of Language*, ed. J. Greenberg (Cambridge, Mass., M.I.T. Press) 53–60.

Fröschels, E.
1915 "Zur behandlung des motorischen aphasie", *Archives Psychiatrist*, 56, 1–19.

Fry, D. B.
1959 "Phonemic substitutions in an aphasic patient", *Language and Speech*, 2, 1, 52–61.

Geschwind, N.
1965a "Disconnexion syndromes in animals and man", I, *Brain*, 88, 2, 237–294.
1965b "Disconnexion syndromes in animals and man", II, *Brain*, 88, 3, 585–644.

Goldstein, K.
1948 *Language and Language Disturbances* (New York, Grune and Stratton).

Goodglass, H., M. Hyde, S. Blumstein
1969 "Frequency, picturability and availability of nouns in aphasia, *Cortex*, 5, 2, 104–119.

Green, E.
1969 "Phonological and grammatical aspects of jargon in an aphasic patient : a case study", *Language and Speech*, 12, 2, 103–118.

Greenberg, J.
1966 "Language universals", in *Current Trends in Linguistics*, III, ed. T. Sebeok (Hague, Mouton) 61–112.

Head, H.
1926 *Aphasia and Kindred Disorders of Speech*, I-II (New York, Hafner).

Hécaen, H. and R. Angelergues
1965 *Pathologie du Langage* (Paris, Larousse).

Howes, D. and N. Geschwind
1964 "Quantitative studies of aphasic language", in *Disorders of Communication*, ed. D. Rioch, E. Weinstein (Baltimore, Williams & Wilkins) 229–244.

Jackson, J. H.
1958 *Selected Writings*, II, ed. J. Taylor, (New York, Basic Books).

Jakobson, R.
1962a "Mufaxxama – the 'emphatic' phonemes in Arabic", in *Roman Jakobson : Selected Writings*, I (Hague : Mouton) 510–522.
1962b "Observations sur le classement phonologique des consonnes," in *Roman Jakobson : Selected Writings*, I (Hague, Mouton) 272–279.
1963a "Implications of language universals for linguistics", in *Universals of Language*, ed. J. Greenberg (Cambridge Mass., M.I.T. Press) 263–278.
1963b "Linguistic types of aphasia", in *Brain Function*, III, ed. E. Carterette, (California, University of California) 67–91.
1964 "Towards a linguistic typology of aphasic impairments", in *Disorders of Language*, ed. A.V.S. de Reuck and M. O'Connor (Boston, Little, Brown) 21–46.
1968 *Child Language, Aphasia, and Phonological Universals*, transl. A.R. Keiler (Hague, Mouton).

Jakobson, R. and M. Halle
1956 *Fundamentals of Language* (Hague, Mouton).

1968 "Phonology in relation to phonetics", *Manual of Phonetics*, ed. B. Malmberg (Amsterdam, North Holland) 411–449.

Jakobson, R., M Halle and G. Fant

1962 *Preliminaries to Speech Analysis* (Cambridge Mass., M.I.T. Press).

Kreindler, A. and A. Fradis

1968 *Performances in Aphasia* (Paris, Gauthier-Villars).

Lecours, A. R. and F. Lhermitte

1969 "Phonemic paraphasias: linguistic structures and tentative hypotheses", *Cortex*, 5, 3, 193–228.

Lehiste, I.

1968 *Some Acoustic Characteristics of Dysarthria* (Switzerland, Biblioteca Phonetica).

Liberman, A.

1961 "Some results of research on speech perception", in *Psycholinguistics*, ed. S. Saporta (New York, Holt, Rinehart & Winston) 142–153.

Lisker, L.

1957 "Minimal cues for separating /w, r, l, y/ in intervocalic position", *Word*, 13, 2, 256–267.

Luria, A. R.

1961 "The pathology of directive function of speech", *Reports at the VIIth International Congress of Neurology*, (Rome) 601–603.

1964 "Factors and forms of aphasia", in *Disorders of Language*, ed. A.V.S. de Reuck and M. O'Connor (Boston, Little, Brown) 143–161.

Ombredane, A.

1926 "Sur le mécanisme de l'anarthrie", *Journal de Psychologie Normale et Pathologique*, 61, 940–955.

Postal, P.

1968 *Aspects of Phonological Theory* (New York, Harper & Row).

Schenk, V. W.

1953 "Troubles des phonèmes en cas d'aphasie sensorielle", *Encéphale*, 42, 158–169.

Shankweiler, D. and K. Harris

1966 "An experimental approach to the problem of articulation in aphasia", *Cortex*, 2, 3, 277–292.

Tarnóczy, T.

1967 "Resonance data concerning nasals, laterals, and trills", in *Readings in Acoustic Phonetics*, ed. I. Lehiste (Cambridge Mass., M.I.T. Press).

Tikofsky, R.

1965 *Phonetic Characteristics of Dysarthria* (Michigan, Office of Research Administration).

Trubetzkoy, N. S.

1958 *Grundzüge der Phonologie* (Gottingen, Vandenhoeck & Ruprecht).

Wepman, J., R. Bock, L. Jones and D. Van Pelt

1956 "Psycholinguistic study of aphasia : a revision of the concept of anomia", *Journal of Speech and Hearing Disorders*, 21, 4, 468–477.

INDEX

JANUA LINGUARUM

STUDIA MEMORIAE NICOLAI VAN WIJK DEDICATA

Edited by C. H. van Schooneveld

SERIES MINOR

42. MILKA IVIĆ: Trends in Linguistics. Translated by Muriel Heppell. 1965. 260 pp. Gld. 28.—
44. THEODORE M. DRANGE: Type Crossings: Sentential Meaninglessness in the Border Area of Linguistics and Philosophy. 1966. 218 pp. Gld. 29.—
45. WARREN H. FAY: Temporal Sequence in the Perception of Speech. 1966. 126 pp., 29 figs. Gld. 23.—
47. BOWMAN CLARKE: Language and Natural Theology. 1966. 181 pp. Gld. 30.—
49. SAMUEL ABRAHAM and FERENC KIEFER: A Theory of Structural Semantics. 1966. 98 pp., 20 figs. Gld. 16.—
50. ROBERT J. SCHOLES: Phonotactic Grammatically. 1966. 117 pp., many figs. Gld. 20.—
51. HOWARD R. POLLIO: The Structural Basis of Word Association Behavior. 1966. 96 pp., 4 folding tables, 8 pp. graphs, figs. Gld. 18.—
52. JEFFREY ELLIS: Towards and General Comparative Linguistics. 1966. 170 pp. Gld. 26.—
54. RANDOLPH QUIRK and JAN SVARTVIK: Investigating Linguistic Acceptability. 1966. 118 pp., 14 figs., 4 tables. Gld. 20.—
55. THOMAS A. SEBEOK (ED.): Selected Writings of Gyula Laziczius. 1966. 226 pp. Gld. 33.—
56. NOAM CHOMSKY: Topics in the Theory of Generative Grammar. 1966. 96 pp. Gld. 12.—
58. LOUIS G. HELLER and JAMES MACRIS: Parametric Linguistics. 1967. 80 pp., 23 tables. Gld. 14.—
59. JOSEPH H. GREENBERG: Language Universals: With Special Reference to Feature Hierarchies. 1966. 89 pp. Gld. 14.—
60. CHARLES F. HOCKETT: Language, Mathematics, and Linguistics. 1967. 244 pp., some figs. Gld. 28.—
62. B. USPENSKY: Principles of Structural Typology. 1968. 80 pp. Gld. 16.—
63. V. Z. PANFILOV: Grammar and Logic. 1968. 160 pp. Gld. 18.—
64. JAMES C. MORRISON: Meaning and Truth in Wittgenstein's Tractatus. 1968. 148 pp. Gld. 20.—
65. ROGER L. BROWN: Wilhelm von Humboldt's Conception of Linguistic Relativity. 1967. 132 pp. Gld. 20.—
66. EUGENE J. BRIERE: A Psycholinguistic Study of Phonological Interference. 1968. 84 pp. Gld. 14.—

67. ROBERT L. MILLER: The Linguistic Relativity Principle and New Humboldtian Ethnolinguistics: A History and Appraisal. 1968. 127 pp. Gld. 20.—
69. I. M. SCHLESINGER: Sentence Structure and the Reading Process. 1968. 172 pp. Gld. 22.—
70. A. ORTIZ and E. ZIERER: Set Theory and Linguistics. 1968. 64 pp. Gld. 12.—
71. HANS-HEINRICH LIEB: Communication Complexes and Their Stages. 1968. 140 pp. Gld. 20.—
72. ROMAN JAKOBSON: Child Language, Aphasia and Phonological Universals. 1968. 104 pp. Gld. 12.—
73. CHARLES F. HOCKETT: The State of the Art. 1968. 124 pp. Gld. 18.—
74. A. JUILLAND and HANS-HEINRICH LIEB: "Klasse" und "Klassifikation" in der Sprachwissenschaft. 1968. 75 pp. Gld. 14.—
76. URSULA OOMEN: Automatische Syntaktische Analyse. 1968. 84 pp. Gld. 16.—
77. ALDO D. SCAGLIONE: Ars Grammatica. 1970. 151 pp. Gld. 18.—
106. HENRIK BIRNBAUM: Problems of Typological and Genetic Linguistics Viewed in a Generative Framework. 1971. 132 pp. Gld. 16.—
107. NOAM CHOMSKY: Studies on Semantics in Generative Grammar. 1972. 207 pp. Gld. 24.—
110. MANFRED BIERWISCH: Modern Linguistics. Its Development, Methods and Problems. 1971. 105 pp. Gld. 12.—
113. ERHARD AGRICOLA: Semantische Relationen im Text und im System. 1972. 127 pp. Gld. 26.—
114. ROMAN JAKOBSON: Studies on Child Language and Aphasia. 1971. 132 pp. Gld. 16.—
117. D. L. OLMSTED: Out of the Mouth of Babes. 1971. 260 pp. Gld. 36.—
119. HERMAN PARRET: Language and Discourse. 1971. 292 pp. Gld. 32.—
123. JOHN W. OLLER: Coding Information in Natural Languages. 1971. 120 pp. Gld. 20.—
134. ROMAN JAKOBSON: A Bibliography of His Writings. With a Foreword by C. H. Van Schooneveld. 1971. 60 pp. Gld. 10.—

MOUTON · PUBLISHERS · THE HAGUE

Bei Fragen zur Produktsicherheit wenden Sie sich bitte an:
If you have any questions regarding product safety,
please contact:

Walter de Gruyter GmbH
Genthiner Straße 13
10785 Berlin
productsafety@degruyterbrill.com